Dyslexia

An Amazing Discovery

by
Jacqui Vittles

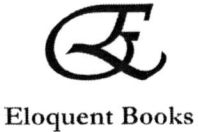

Eloquent Books

Eloquent Books
An imprint of Strategic Book Group
P.O. Box 333
Durham CT 06422
www.StrategicBookGroup.com

ISBN: 978-1-60860-843-0

Printed in the United States of America

Book Design: Suzanne Kelly

This book is dedicated to all those people yet to discover their gift, and to all those who live or work with them.

Thanks

I give my humble and heartfelt gratitude to my husband, who remains a constant source of inspiration and support for my efforts; to my sons, for their patience, generosity and for believing in me; to Ali, Pavel, Phil, Phil, Cris, Grant, Jo, Robin, Penelope and Lynn for their invaluable contributions and constant encouragement; to Joy for keeping my fingers tapping on the keys and guiding me through the morass; and to Irina, who sowed the seed that got me to commit my story to paper in the first place.

I give my humble and heartfelt apologies to anyone who ever asked me to read a text book—and expected me to learn something from it!

Dyslexia

An Amazing Discovery

Contents

About This Book

This book is not about dyslexia. This book is about my experience of being dyslexic and not knowing. It is about my personal journey struggling without realising it and how I came to discover what was—or wasn't—actually *wrong* with me. Having already held down high-powered management jobs, gained an MBA and run my own business, I made the life-changing discovery. It felt like emerging from a dark tunnel into the light for the very first time.

As I now know, dyslexia is a much-misunderstood condition. For a start, it isn't an illness that can be cured and therefore it doesn't have medical symptoms. What it does have is a series of characteristics that can be both inconsistent and challenging. The term *word-blindness* is often used as short-hand for describing the condition, but as I discovered, this is misleading. In fact, it represents only a fraction of those characteristics that join together to form the condition we know as dyslexia. Although I have displayed many of those characteristics throughout my life, traditional word-blindness has never really been one of them. I am also of above-average intelligence and these two factors together militated against my discovering that my *little problems* have a name—until I was in the latter half of my forties.

I am not an expert in the condition of dyslexia but I am expert in my own experience of it. My primary motivation in writing this book is in helping others, like myself, to put a name to something they've been aware of all their lives. In sharing my experiences in this way I'm also hoping that people who do not have dyslexia may increase their understanding of what it is and how it can affect other people who may be very close to them.

As well as looking at my own experience of the condition, I have also listened to other people with dyslexia and learnt a great deal more from hearing their stories; and I have discovered that some very famous people are dyslexic, or were during their lifetime. Finally, I have included some information about where readers might be able to go for help if this book has had some resonance for them.

We are learning more and more about dyslexia with each passing year and having the condition is nothing to be ashamed of or hidden away. I hope you enjoy reading this book. If you feel so inclined, please recommend it to someone else who may be interested in this complex and widely misunderstood condition and who may, in turn, go on to share a newfound understanding with others.

The Discovery

My husband Paul and I would often wander into town on a Saturday and have a browse through the bookshops. Paul would always head for the management and motivation sections while I would usually have a look through the sales tables or the display stands with the new releases and books on special promotion, then we'd go for a coffee before making our way back home again.

This particular Saturday was no different. Paul made his way to his favourite section while I ambled towards a table piled high with books on special offer. On one corner of the table was a stack of books about how to train your recalcitrant dog not to chew your furniture, and next to that was a large tome extolling the delights of Chinese cooking for people with no time to cook. I was being invited to brush-up my French in five easy stages and advice on making the best of my somewhat middle-aged looks was jockeying for position with guidance on successfully completing a new, quick and easy ten-point detox plan. Sitting proudly in the centre was a huge pile of autobiographies by someone with an unpronounceable name whom, clearly, no-one wanted to read about. Then, tucked away, partially obscured by our erstwhile luminary, I spotted a medium-sized paperback book sporting a black, white and red cover which announced 'The Gift of Dyslexia'.

I was intrigued as to how dyslexia could be described as a *gift* and picked up the book, almost as a reflex action. I knew there had been studies linking dyslexia with young people with behavioural problems, and I also knew there was anecdotal evidence to suggest that dyslexia is present in a significant proportion of the prison population. I had always believed dyslexia to be a learning disability found particularly amongst people with low IQ and had never really given it a lot of thought beyond these scant few details.

On impulse, I began to read the book. This was most unusual because of my discomfort in reading in a public place, albeit to myself. It was as if the book was willing me to read it. The pages were drawing me to them, beginning with a simple list of the *abilities* that dyslexics share. I saw *highly intuitive* and *perceptive* and I thought, yes, I can identify with that. Being able to think using all the senses. Thinking in pictures … doesn't everyone? Vivid imagination. All these things, the book told me, add up to non-verbal thought. The opposite is linear thought, which is the way language is structured and the way we learn, using sequences and lists. Some pages whispered to me, some shouted at me. They all said something that struck a chord for me.

I stopped reading and looked up. All around me, people were going about their business oblivious of the miracle that was unfolding there, before them, in the middle of that bookshop. Slowly, I raised the book and resumed my reading. My mind flashed a picture of an Alice in Wonderland room with doors lining the walls. The doors opened as I looked at them and bright lights shone from the rooms behind. I relaxed my shoulders as a wave of euphoria washed over me. With a huge sense of relief and a beaming smile, I realised I'm not lazy, I'm not dim or stupid ... I'm *dyslexic*!

I was 46 and I felt the weight of the world lifting from my shoulders. The final piece of life's jigsaw puzzle had gently fallen into place. I no longer had to search for excuses because I had an *explanation*. I'd had no idea that my *little problem* had a name. Not only was I not stupid, I was a *genius* for getting this far, unknowingly developing complex and effective coping strategies that had allowed me to function in a world that people without dyslexia take in their stride. I had positively thrived, against all the odds. As I stood in the middle of the bookshop with all the world going about its business, I realised there's nothing wrong with my brain; it's just wired differently so that information is processed in a different way. All these years I've had to *reprocess* life's information, turning it into a form that I can understand.

I stood, motionless, amid a sea of activity. I breathed deeply and tears welled up in my eyes as my husband ambled towards me with an armful of books on his way to the checkout. Speechless, I simply put *my* book on the top of the pile and smiled at his puzzled expression. Explanations could wait. I was enjoying the precious moment.

Keep the Kettle Boiling

The youngest of three daughters, I was born into a family in the North East of England where I spent the first seventeen years of my life. By most accounts, it was a very normal childhood. I went to a good school, I did ballet classes and enjoyed sports. My parents stayed together in a loving relationship until my mother's death, by which time they had celebrated their Golden wedding anniversary.

As the youngest child, some would say I was indulged although I would not agree. I had a sunny disposition, wavy ginger hair, a cute little snub nose and spoke with a slight lisp. I was a healthy and physically active child with a very vivid imagination. I loved nothing more than to listen to stories—and to make them up.

When I started school, my parents were told that I was a lively and intelligent child although it was also suggested that I had poor concentration and didn't seem to like to sit down and learn, preferring to pick and choose the things to which I wanted to pay attention.

I can still recall my very first day at school. Having two elder sisters, I knew something of the routine of having to wear a uniform, to be at school for a certain time and to bring home things that you had to learn. Mammy told me it was all part of being a 'big girl' and growing up. I couldn't wait to get started.

As I walked through the front door of the school with my mammy I was struck by a new kind of smell. The smell of books, pencils and paper, of erasers and poster paints and all those other things to be found in a school stationery cupboard. Although the smell was not unique to that school, it was my first encounter with it and it is one that can, even now, conjure up some very mixed emotions for me. I loved it then, and still do, but it can also make the hairs on the back of my neck stand on end because of its association with longing to be praised for getting things right and total frustration at consistently getting things wrong.

Just inside the front door was a short corridor which opened out into a communal hallway. All around the walls were the pegs we were to use for our coats and hats. Each peg had a picture next to it and I chose the one with a ship on it, because my daddy had been a marine engineer before he and mammy were married. At about knee height, running along the wall below the pegs, was a long bench we could sit on to change into our indoor shoes and below the bench was a series of wire cubbies in which we could store our outdoor shoes.

I felt so proud, smiling beatifically in my new school uniform. I had been pestering mammy for days to let me wear it, but she had not given in so, there I was, fully adorned for the first time. My ginger curls peaked out from under my little grey felt hat which was held in place by elastic running under my chin. The brim was turned up and my new school badge was proudly aligned over my forehead, sewn onto a navy blue band running all the way around and with a flat bow positioned somewhere around my left ear. Under my navy blue gabardine raincoat, I wore a little grey blazer—slightly too big for me, but bought to grow into—with the school badge sewn onto the breast pocket. It had two large patch pockets, one of which had a clean hanky tucked away neatly in the corner. I wore a regulation pale blue blouse with a peter pan collar and over that was a grey, v-neck jumper. Matching my jumper was a little grey knitted kilt that was held up by knitted braces which snuggled beneath my jumper and over my blouse, making a capital H shape at the front. I knew it was an H because my big sister's name was Heather and that's how her name started. Mammy put my gym bag over my peg and helped me off with my coat and hat. She sat me down on the bench and helped me put on my indoor shoes then tucked my outdoor shoes into my cubby.

Miss Marks, my first teacher, was a tall, slender lady who reminded me of a grandma because she had grey hair, although she didn't look like *my* grandma. She wore square, wire-framed glasses, a neatly ironed blouse with little embroidery flowers on the collar, a matching cardigan and a pleated tweed skirt. The most striking thing my childish eyes noticed was how her bottom teeth went in a curved line, upwards, and her top teeth seemed to be in a curved line, upwards, to match them. This looked odd because most people's teeth met in the middle, in a straight line, with two front teeth bigger than the others, but Miss Marks' were smaller and squashed-looking. She was a gently spoken woman who never seemed to need to raise her voice and, although dealing with all the mothers very respectfully, handled them as if they were a tiresome intrusion to her otherwise very orderly classroom. She smelled of Hyacinths.

My first classroom was light and airy and filled with small tables, each painted bright, daffodil yellow and with a drawer sporting a little red knob in the middle. Miss Marks explained that this drawer was for anything we had brought from home but didn't need in the classroom. Anything that was too big for the drawer had to be either hung on our peg in the cloakroom or put into our shoe-cubby below our peg. I chose a table close to the door which, although I had no idea would be the case at the time, turned out to be highly significant and denoted the first step on my path towards an increased sense of frustration at being trapped within the school environment. I waved goodbye to my mammy and watched, bewildered, as other children clung, weeping and wailing, onto theirs. I wondered if I was supposed to cry, but decided against it.

A window ran the full length of the wall opposite the door and along this window wall was a series of playing areas that included a Wendy House complete with fully fitted kitchen and brightly painted plaster food—I can still recall the smell of the varnish covering those neat little cakes and vegetables—a table with four, three-legged stools and a tiny play bed next to a little window with green gingham curtains that could be pulled closed. Along the wall running at right-angles to the windows was a shiny red slide with six or seven rungs on the ladder leading to the top. In front of that was a blue and red two-seater roundabout that was worked by each child having a lever to pull backwards and forwards. Standing in the corner was a tall wooden easel with two legs at the front and one at the back, connected by a length of grey rope. There was a series of holes running up the two front legs and a wooden peg in each leg held a very large blackboard in place.

Along the wall opposite the windows was a series of small shelves with paper, pens, games and brightly coloured wooden toys. Above these were display boards with lots of bright, colourful pictures. Miss Marks' desk and chair were along this wall and I was to become very familiar with observing the activities in the room from this perspective. The wall running at right-angles to the other end of the window wall had lots of posters with letters on. Then there was a series of large blue cards with bright red dots on, each one with a corresponding number below it. My little five-year old eyes took in the scene with great wonderment and longing.

. . .

During that first year we used to play a game called 'Keep the Kettle Boiling' which was a very simple concept and a great motivator—for some. Miss Marks would write a series of sums on the blackboard and we had to copy each one down in our little exercise books. Once you'd copied one down, worked out and written down the answer, shown it to the teacher and got a lovely red tick next to it, you could have a go on the slide then go back to your seat and copy down the next one. And so it went on until you had done all the sums on the board, then you could either keep going down the slide or play in the Wendy House until everyone had finished.

The first time we played it, I took my turn waiting in line at Miss Marks' desk, only to see a red cross appear next to my best efforts and then be told to go back and try again. This sequence happened several times until I hit on the idea of copying my friend Jane's answer. She'd already been down the slide several times and it seemed to me like a very sensible way to solve my problem. Sure enough, this time I got a beautiful red tick and off I went, proudly climbing up the rungs and sliding gracefully down to the bottom of the shiny red slide. Unfortunately, sometime between receiving my red tick and arriving at the bottom of the slide, Miss Marks discovered that I had not been altogether honest about my efforts and I was severely reprimanded. It is my first recollection of the kind of toe-curling humiliation that I was to become very familiar with.

Number work was a constant bafflement, although I loved visualising shapes and colours, playing in my mind's eye with the patterns that were formed by the dots on the giant domino cards. To this day, I love the formation of five as a dot in each corner and one in the middle. But learning anything by rote was a complete waste of time and I can honestly say, with my hand on my heart, I *still* don't know my multiplication tables. I can work them out through a combination of visualising multiple doubles and recreating the various shapes I associate with certain numbers, but as for actually knowing the *sequence* of numbers—it still eludes me.

I was also slow in learning to read and was always amongst the small group who had to go to 'the room with the blue table cloth', as it was called, to have extra sessions for my reading. This was a very quiet room, lined with filing cabinets and shelves, with a very large, stolid table in the centre that reached up to my neck height. The blue table cloth covering the table resembled the kind of willow-pattern plates that my grandma said she used to keep 'for best' and I would be eye-to-eye with the embossed patterns formed from the woven linen threads. I felt completely intimidated by the silence—broken only by a ticking clock—and by the expectation of the teacher waiting to hear me read, hesitantly and falteringly from my reading book. I remember very little from these sessions to do with reading, but I do recall feeling nauseous and sweaty, and the sting in my eyes as the tears began to well up. There is no way on this earth I could have put into words the sheer frustration of wanting *so hard* to get it right but failing miserably to achieve it. I wanted to be told I was a 'clever girl'—what child wouldn't?—but what I repeatedly experienced was a palpable sense of disappointment from my teacher. My ears buzzed and the tears welled up, despite my best efforts, and only served to make my teacher—and my mammy and daddy—more annoyed with me. 'We know you can be a good girl, Jacqui, if only you would work hard and concentrate'.

Needless to say, my favourite time of day was play time and I would always long to be outside, but I was often held back in the classroom to finish off my work before I was allowed to go out and join my classmates—if there was time.

'Listen carefully!' 'You're daydreaming!' 'Pay attention now, Jacqui!' Patiently and not-so-patiently I was cajoled and coaxed into learning the things it was deemed I needed to know, in order to receive a good education. 'You must concentrate hard because I know you can get it right when you do'.

. . .

Through those early years I was a bright and lively member of my class but sitting at my allotted desk held little attraction for me. I would look at a picture in a book or on the wall, or even from my own imaginings, and my child's mind would carry me off into another world, playing out a story with real characters and animals and colours. Then I'd find myself being told to go back to my own seat and get on with my work. Unfortunately, when the instructions had been given by the teacher I was absent, in my other world, and I would have no idea what I was supposed to be doing. Wanting to work hard and be a good girl, I didn't like to ask what to do because then I would be told I should have been listening and my teacher would be cross with me. I had learnt that I mustn't copy other people's work and so, more often than not, my page would remain empty or filled with things that were irrelevant to the task in hand.

My second teacher in those infant years was a small, slim woman called Mrs Taylor. She was younger than Miss Marks and wore black framed glasses which turned upwards at the sides, as was the fashion in the late 1950s. She had short wavy hair which was just starting to grey at the temples and wore neat jumpers with fitted skirts and low-heeled shoes. I'm not sure if it is simply my impression from this far removed but my recollection is that her clothes were always shades of grey.

My classroom at that time also seemed to be dark, which was quite a contrast to the light and airy room that was now next door. All the desks were old, varnished wood and had a lid that lifted up with a space beneath for storing our books and pencils. The lid was angled slightly downwards with a long metal hinge along each side and a groove on the top for resting our pencils in when we weren't writing with them. Mrs Taylor's desk was raised up on a low platform at the front of the room and next to it was a large blackboard on an easel.

In the corner of the room was a door that led into our cloakroom. I remember very little about the arrangements here and can bring only a scant visual picture to mind, other than one occasion when I was not able to untangle the knot in one of my shoe laces. All my friends had gone into the classroom and I was left on my own, with only my hot stinging tears for company. The bleary vision my tears caused didn't help me resolve the situation and I recall bruising the top of my foot as I forced it out of my shoe.

Even at this young age, I knew Mrs Taylor didn't like me because most of the time she simply ignored me. I wanted to be in the group of clever girls with Sarah and Fiona and Katherine and so I would try my hardest to draw her attention. But this never seemed to work. In fact it made her sigh, impatiently … and so I tried harder. What I didn't realise was that it was precisely my behaviour in trying to draw her attention that was fuelling her dislike … but I just wanted to be a good girl, so I kept trying harder and harder.

The pattern of behaviour that began here was to be repeated many times throughout my school years and, indeed, into adulthood. I would listen to chatter and talk that was going on around me but, often, could not find the right words to engage with others and involve myself in what was being said. When I was excited or tired my words would come out back-to-front or with part of the phonetic missing. I could *feel* what I wanted to say and could, somehow, visualise a shape or form for it, but I couldn't actually say the words. This led to more frustration both on my part, because I couldn't say what I wanted to say, and on my teacher's part because she thought I was just being lazy, or cheeky, or rude. This was exacerbated further because the problem was intermittent. There would be many occasions when I was relaxed and calm, where I could speak fluently but those occasions when I couldn't would be accompanied by the churning feeling in the pit of my stomach, a sweaty sensation down my back, the customary gripping of my toes inside my shoes and, yes, those ubiquitous hot, stinging tears.

I have been gifted with the capacity to see the bigger picture in most situations I encounter and to evaluate situations very quickly and intuitively. As an adult, this can be a very effective tool when negotiating life's ups and downs but, as a child, this was very troublesome because I didn't know it for what it was. As a child, this capacity translated into pure bossiness which was alienating to all around, particularly because I wasn't able to articulate those things that I *felt* so instinctively. I could always work out, very quickly, what would be a good plan but I couldn't say *why* it was a good plan ... I just insisted that it was. As a result, I alienated myself from my peers and was always the last to be chosen for any group activities because my classmates all knew I would either be bossy, or I would cry.

. . .

As I moved up through my infant school years and into the junior classes, these same patterns became more and more developed. What was missing now, however, was the cute little ginger curly-haired girl who had accompanied the behaviour and masked some of the more unpleasant traits. As I grew up, 'you should know better' started to become the new response from others.

I was always completely absorbed in any projects that involved arts and crafts and although I was never particularly dexterous—another source of frustration to my teachers—I loved making things, especially if it gave me an opportunity to get up and move around the classroom. I recall spending what appeared to be many laborious hours poring over the construction of a glove puppet made from felt, with a papier-maché head. We had to blanket stitch the seams of the body together, which caused me no end of problems and led, in the end, to my designing a new kind of stitch. The head was created by gluing layers and layers of small pieces of newspaper to the outside of a small balloon, building a protrusion for a nose and creating dents for the eye sockets. When the paper was dry, we burst the balloon leaving a hollow shape which was then painted to create the features of the face. A piece of empty toilet roll was pushed up into the hole to form a neck and that was where our fingers went, when our hands were inside the felt body.

Mine was a witch. I had created a long hooked nose and a big chin which curved upwards to meet it. I gave it one tooth and painted the rest of the inside of the mouth, black. I cut several short strands of black wool and stuck them on the top the head, to create hair. It was ugly. The effect was striking and this creation was my pride and joy. I can still smell the varnish that we used to coat the finished product.

It was when I was in Miss Laws' class that we had been engaged in this craft project and not long after completing it we had a reading test. Miss Laws was my most favourite teacher of all time. She was very young. Her hair flicked upwards at the bottom and she wore bright red lipstick. She carried a wicker basket to school every day that was always filled with books. She wore a heavy, olive green coat which had a large roll-neck collar and was fastened at the side with one button. It was the largest button I had ever seen.

Miss Laws lived quite close to where I lived and sometimes I would walk along with her. I loved Miss Laws. She was kind. She didn't ignore me and listened as I told her all my stories— mostly grounded in truth, somewhere along the way, but greatly embellished for the benefit of my audience.

When Miss Laws announced the reading test, everyone groaned … as young children do. She told us there would be three parts to it. Firstly we would have to read out single words that she showed us from a list, then we would have a short piece to read that we hadn't seen before, but then we could read something of our own choice that we had read before. It could be anything we wanted, from any of our books at home or at school. I didn't have many books at home but there was a book I'd been given at Christmas which included a story about a witch. This was the one for me and I loved Miss Laws so much I wanted to read it really well for her … so I learned it by heart, word for word. And just for good measure, I practiced a croaky witch's voice for the bits where the witch was speaking.

Miss Laws was thrilled with my efforts. She congratulated me heartily on an excellent achievement and, for the first time in my life, gave me a Highly Commended mark for my test—despite not doing very well with the words list and the unseen reading. I was positively glowing with pride and skipped all the way home to tell my mammy I had been a 'clever girl'. I knew she would be very pleased with me, and indeed she was. I was rewarded with a big hug, but her words came ringing in my ears, 'you see, all you have to do is try hard and you do well. We know you can do it. Now let's see if you can do this every time from now on'.

This was a perfectly reasonable sentiment but, although I would not have known the saying at the time, I had well and truly shot myself in the foot. My very best efforts to be a clever girl had, in fact, conspired against me and would come back to haunt me, time and time again.

Pins and Needles

It was in Mrs Elliot's class that we started to learn how to do joined-up writing. I recall very little about my earlier efforts in learning to write my letters of the alphabet, which probably reflects the fact that I would avoid it at all costs. The problem of inverting my *p*'s and *q*'s and my *d*'s and *b*'s seemed to pose no greater problem for me than for many other children sitting around me in my class. My *k*'s would sometimes present themselves backwards and I recall spending quite some time looking at pictures of *curly c* and *kicking k*. My *s*'s often snaked the wrong way, but other than that, my learning process—albeit painfully slow—was reasonably accurate. But then we moved into Mrs Elliot's class and started the serious business of proper writing, which was an altogether different story.

The classrooms for the junior children were on the first floor of the big old house that formed my school in those early years. It was in these classrooms that Mrs Elliot told us we were to become 'big girls' and more would be expected of us. We were told we had to set an example for the younger girls by concentrating hard, behaving properly and doing good work. I bought this mantra in its entirety because I wanted Mrs Elliot to be pleased with me and for her to acknowledge and praise my efforts.

Mrs Elliot often used to read to us and she introduced us to the stories of Worzel Gummidge, which I adored. As she was reading I would be transported into my *other world* and could see the characters as if they were real, playing out their story in front of me. The only problem was that we were expected to be reading it at home at the same time but, somehow, I never quite got around to reading it at home and was often caught out if we had to answer questions about any part of the story Mrs Elliot had not yet read.

Mrs Elliot was a small, bustley kind of lady who would regularly fuss about things. She was short and very round. She wore tight-fitting, woollen hounds-tooth checked skirts and had spectacles on a chain around her neck. She had milky blue, slightly bulging eyes and neat, greying, tight-curled hair through which she would regularly run her fingers. Everywhere Mrs Elliot went, she carried a voluminous handbag into which she would often dive to retrieve a scrunched bag of boiled sweets then surreptitiously pop one into her mouth. She would perch her spectacles on the end of her nose when she was concentrating on something in front of her, then whip them off again when she looked up to speak to us. This had the resultant effect of making the spectacles appear to be on short elastic as they bounced, continuously, up and down from her nose to her ample bosom and back up to her nose again.

All Mrs Elliot's favourite girls were placed in the two rows at the front, around her desk and it was to these girls that most of our lessons were given. My desk was in the row second from back. I seldom received a 'good work' from Mrs Elliot and have little recollection of any comments from her other than a regular, impatiently spluttered, 'Hurry up now, Jacqui. You're holding everyone up'.

Joining up my letters caused me great difficulty. By now, I had mastered the art of getting my letters round the right way and was reasonably proficient at choosing the right letters to put together to make the right sound, like *ee* or *ea* or *oo* etc. Joining them all together, though, was a task that consistently defeated me. But this was such an important task that Miss Marks—who Mrs Elliot described as, 'the most important teacher in our school'—came upstairs especially to teach us. I'm not sure what effect this was supposed to have on us but, unfortunately, it terrified me. For some reason, my pen never went back to the same place after I'd lifted it off the paper, making it look as if a family of spiders had been throwing a party. And then there was my little trick of missing words out, or writing them again, when I'd already written them—wasn't one lot of torture enough? You would think I'd notice that I'd done it but, somehow, I never did until it was pointed out by Miss Marks, with her customary sigh. 'I do wish you'd concentrate, Jacqui' was usually muttered as she moved on to the next girl.

On one memorable occasion, Miss Marks came upstairs for our writing session and informed us that this was a very important letter that was to be copied from the blackboard and taken home to give to our parents. If I was terrified during the normal sessions, this piece of information made my brain freeze over completely and from that moment on, all I could hear was a dull buzzing in my ears as my toes crunched up in my shoes and my sweaty little fingers gripped my freshly sharpened pencil. I could see Miss Marks pointing at the blackboard and I could see her mouth opening and closing, but my brain had left the room and was already populating another universe somewhere, anywhere, other than the room my body was in.

Before my mental escape, she had told us that we were to write an invitation to our school Sports Day and carefully gave us all a sheet of what she called, 'special paper'. She gave us only one sheet each and warned us not to make any mistakes. She told us how to measure down both sides of the paper and where to put little tiny dots, then draw a line across the sheet to join up the two marks, nice and lightly with our pencil, along the edge of our ruler. These were the lines where we had to write our words, so it would keep our writing neat and straight. I began to feel pins and needles in my bottom, as if the seat of my chair was on fire, which made me jiggle from side to side. It was soon after this that my brain went on its walkabout but after a while I was brought back into the room with a thump when I heard Miss Marks ask the class how we were getting on and to put our hands up if we needed anything. I looked down at my sheet of paper which was devoid of lines and letters, joined-up or otherwise but I wanted so much to engage with Miss Marks and for her to be pleased with me that I recalled how Miss Laws used to like us to tell her our news, and I put my hand up.

Miss Marks looked up and noticed my hand. She got up slowly from behind her desk and walked up to the back of the classroom where I was sitting.

'Yes, Jacqui. What is it?' she asked very purposefully, accompanied by the withering look with which I was becoming all too familiar.

'Miss Marks', I began, 'The Sports Day is on 6th July and that's the day my Auntie's having her baby'. Blank look from Miss Marks. 'My Auntie used to come to this school', I offered, perhaps hoping it would be some recompense for not having a question about the task in hand—and indeed, for having nothing written on my special piece of paper. I knew Miss Laws would have been delighted with this news and would probably have asked me to tell her some more about it. Miss Marks, on the other hand, continued to look blankly at me then simply said, 'Your page is empty, Jacqui. Get on with your work, please', before slowly turning on her heels, walking back to her desk and replacing her long frame onto her seat.

The buzzing returned and this time it was accompanied by the old familiar sick-feeling in the pit of my stomach. The stinging in my eyes was pulsing in unison with the curling of my toes and I just sat, completely motionless, until the bell sounded for playtime. Miss Marks stood up and gathered her papers together as all my classmates went out to play. She took the blackboard duster and wiped off the words everyone—except me, that is— had copied onto their special sheets of paper. She put the cleaner back onto its ledge, picked up her papers and quietly walked out of the classroom. I was still there when everyone came back in at the end of playtime and Mrs Elliot, complete with voluminous handbag and boiled sweets, joined us for storytime.

My mammy and daddy didn't come to Sports Day that year but it was the year I won the Obstacle Race.

. . .

I think it was around this time that I really began to develop a keen sense of envy. My greatest need was to be praised, but I never was. Instead, I became acutely aware of all the girls around me who were doing good work, getting it right and being praised for it, and through this the seeds of envy were sown. I was acutely embarrassed by my handwriting, joined-up or otherwise. I wanted to write neatly, just like Miss Marks and Mrs Elliot wanted me to, but my handwriting was a mess and so I hid it, avoided it, scribbled over it in frustration—anything that would release me from the torment. Everyone around me had beautiful handwriting and never made any mistakes— or so it seemed—and I sat at my desk, in my own little world, dreaming about having beautiful handwriting but staring down at the evidence of my nightmare. If wishes were currency—I would have been a very rich little girl.

I think it was also around this time that my morbid fear of numbers really started to kick in. I had had problems from the start, recognising values and relating them to the figure that was written down. Seeing the values as dots helped but, ultimately, the lines and curves I was required to draw had no meaning. I couldn't relate them to anything and so instead I sat dreaming of the shapes they formed. Sometimes, I even got my coloured pencils out and made pictures with the shapes formed around the lines. I loved the formation of the number five, represented by a dot in four corners and one in the middle, but I could not write the figure 5. It defeated me. But even writing this figure was easier then writing a number 8— which I still have problems with. Over and over again, I was expected to start at the top left, go downwards to the right, curve around the bottom, up to the top right and back around the top to join up with where I'd started—but could I do it? Over and over again, I couldn't. Some form of impulse stopped me from being able to create the number. I couldn't *see* it. I couldn't follow the pattern with my pencil. I couldn't follow the pattern with my eyes. I still start my 8's at the bottom right and it's a miracle if it ever joins back up again where I started.

We were introduced to hundreds, tens, and units, but it may as well have been jam, treacle and rice pudding for all I could understand it. And when we began to write down multiplication and division sums I was completely and utterly defeated. I was shown the physical quantities of something and was asked to divide or multiply them, and I had no problem understanding the concept but I just couldn't write it down or make sense of it all on paper.

'Now come along, Jacqui, concentrate. You've just shown me the answer with your beans and now all you have to do is write it down on your paper, like I've shown you'. Easy!

It never occurred to me that other people might *see* numbers differently to me. From my very earliest recollections, odd numbers, as opposed to even numbers, have terrified me, and I use that word deliberately. They're not balanced. There's a bit missing. They're jagged around the edges and you have to be careful of the pointy bits. In particular, the number 17 brings cold shivers down my spine. I find myself physically—although not visibly—repulsed by it. 'Uh-oh', I instinctively think to myself, 'Here comes trouble!' It's brown and angular. It doesn't fit. The number 19, although still brown, has four corners but each side is a different length. The number 19 takes my breath away, as if I've been running uphill with it towards the number 20, but not quite made it. The number 21 has just gone too far. If 20 is on a platform, 21 has just fallen off the side, to the right.

But for some reason, the number five rings true for me. I love it. It was the first multiplication table I ever learnt. It's completely balanced, being absolutely half way between nothing and 10, 10 and 20, 20 and 30 and so on. Five makes me feel warm and comfortable, and never lets me down. It smiles at me. It makes me feel confident … unless I have to write it down, of course.

As an adult, I just accept all this and take it in my stride. As a child, not realising that other people couldn't see what I could see, I couldn't understand why I couldn't understand. I would stare at my paper and *will* the sums to give me the right answers. I had learnt, the hard way, not to copy from the girls sitting around me and would try my hardest to write down what my teacher wanted me to write—but it wouldn't come.

'Jacqui is an intelligent little girl, but she must try harder and concentrate on her work' was the most often repeated comment on my report card at the end of each school term. It's no wonder my parents were exasperated with me—and it's no wonder I started to become resentful and envious. And this was when I started to feel an acute sense of guilt. Everyone wanted me to do better and I was just letting them down, all the time.

· · ·

Receiving all new information in *pictures* is something that has always been the norm for me and, as a little girl, I simply assumed this was the same for everyone.

I had great problems learning how to tell the time because I couldn't visualise it. Mammy and daddy assigned my big sister, Heather, to teaching me how to tell the time and I recall spending what seemed like hours on hands and knees on our dining room floor, moving the red hands around a large, black-and-white cardboard clockface. The o'clocks were easy, as was half-past. Quarter-to and quarter-past took a little longer, but I got the hang of it eventually. The problems really kicked in when it came to understanding the other positions for the long hand ... and the concept of the short hand, pointing to the hours of the day. Time and time again it defeated me but it's a testament to my sister's patience (she was to become a teacher of children with special needs) that I did, eventually learn to tell the time.

I also duly learnt the days of the week, as did all the little girls around me, and could tell the teacher what day it was, and even the month—eventually. But how many of my little friends were seeing what I saw?

To pause in the chronology of my story for a moment, let me ask you, for example, how you *see* a week? When someone says to you, 'It'll take a week for it to come through' or perhaps, 'The Festival lasted for a week', what do you see? I discuss this with friends, now, and they tell me they don't *see* anything. If pushed, they'll tell me they can visualise a diary, or perhaps a calendar of the type you may hang on the wall where the days are laid out in sequence and there are spaces to mark in particular events, or birthdays, etc.

When this is described to me I too can see it this way, but what I first see when thinking of a week is a long, angular line resembling the shape of a castle wall, with turrets. Saturday and Sunday are high up in a horizontal line, then there's a straight vertical drop to

Monday, followed horizontally by Tuesday. Wednesday pops upwards again to form a short horizontal line, but not to the same height as Saturday and Sunday. There's another vertical drop to Thursday but this is lower than Monday and Tuesday. Friday joins with Thursday, but together their horizontal line is longer than Monday and Tuesday's. At the end of this, Saturday and Sunday return to stand together on a high horizontal platform. Can you see the castle wall in this description?

Critically, however, this visual line actually runs backwards for me, from right to left, and I see it in a split-second of time.

And, how do you *see* a calendar year? I see a shape similar to a rugby ball, but less clearly defined. December is grey and starts at the left point with the dark (I was born in the Northern Hemisphere) months running long and low towards the right. April forms a small interlude of green and yellow, and appears to me as if I was on a train which stops in the countryside for a short while. June (my birth month) is pinky-red and leads the way into a new direction, and the light months arc upwards and back along to the left. September is turning brown and getting dark again, October is white and November (darkish green) slopes back down to meet December. Again, all visualised within a split-second.

Confused? As a little girl, this is what a week and a year was to me. This is what I thought everyone could see.

. . .

When I was eight years old, we were offered extra classes at our school, outside of the normal school timetable. My mum was told that I had, 'a neat and compact physique that might lend itself to ballet classes'—and so I duly started Friday afternoon ballet. I loved it. I was in my element. At last I could do something that brought smiles to the faces of my teacher and my mammy and daddy.

'Oh, that's very nice, Jacqui', was met with a huge grin and blushing cheeks. It wasn't something I was used to hearing and, in some strange way, it made me feel uncomfortable. I loved to hear it, and it made me point my toes even harder and jump even higher—but there was that small part of me that didn't believe it. And anyway, it was only ballet. It wasn't *real* work, was it?

My friend Barbara and I became famed for our polka. We were the only ones who could get the rhythm right and we polkaed our way around the dance floor at the end of term demonstration. I was so happy and so was Miss Cromarty, our teacher. I wanted my teachers to continue to tell me what a clever girl I was but, sadly, once I got back to the classroom, it all evaporated and I was back to the anguish, the squirming and the pins and needles in my bottom.

'Now come along, Jacqui. Concentrate on your work and you'll soon be able to go out to play'. It was a great incentive but ... concentrate on what? If whatever it was I was learning about hadn't appeared to me visually, it simply didn't register. If my teachers could explain it to me in a way I could visualise, I could grasp the concept and could answer questions about it. But the older I got, the more we were required to read and learn from text books ... and this just became one more mountain to climb.

The one respite from my mathematical mountain was geometry ... and I loved it. I enjoyed working out the size of an angle in a triangle, or memorizing the names for the different kinds of shapes, according to how many sides they had. I understood about circumferences and diameters, although I wasn't too good at working out the lengths of these. Miss Brown simply couldn't understand how I could do good work with geometry when all the rest of my arithmetic was so abysmal. Here was one more example of Jacqui shooting herself in the foot. How could I be good at one thing and so bad at another, related thing? Answer: because I wasn't concentrating hard enough. In the eyes of my teachers and my parents,

I was intelligent and capable of doing good work … when I wanted to. All I had to do was put my mind to it but, 'for some reason, Jacqui, you choose not to!'

I took comfort in being good at my ballet, which by now had led me to extra classes outside of school, but I so longed to be clever at school. I so longed to have neat writing and I so longed to be able to get my sums right. I so longed to be able to speak and answer questions, coherently, and I so longed to be able to pass my exams with ease. As my envy grew, so did my resentment. As my sense of guilt grew, so did my aggressive self-defence and my tendency to say 'it's not my fault', which, quite understandably, was always met with, 'well, whose fault is it then?' I know now that it's an impossible question to answer because it is, actually, no-one's fault. If only I'd known then.

Brains in My Feet

Around about the same time that my hormones were beginning to catapult me into adolescence and the telltale characteristics of envy, guilt and a feisty attitude really started to take form, my class graduated up into the senior school which was another old building up the hill and across the road from the prep school I had been attending.

In my adult life, a friend once suggested that adolescence is a social construct. Up until around 50 years ago, a boy grew up and at a certain age began to dress and behave like his father. Likewise a girl would have her rite of passage into womanhood. A girl had to learn how to cook and sew and keep house. She was also expected to want to find a good man to marry and to have babies. Puberty, whether for a boy or a girl, was something to be endured and was never spoken of. It signalled the coming of the end of childhood and a progression into adulthood.

By the time I reached the age when hormones were raging through my body, that social construct was in full swing. The Beatles had arrived and my adolescence was beginning to make its presence felt. I took to it very comfortably in my customary, precocious manner. Having two elder sisters certainly helped me to develop into a state of longing to be grown up, long before I had developed the physical, psychological or emotional toolkit to deal with it. All the usual signs of burgeoning womanhood could not come fast enough for me. The acne and the oily hair were the less pleasant indicators that I was on my way. The erstwhile pimples on my chest were now starting to sprout and soft, curly hair was starting to cover the parts that, bare, would otherwise indicate I was still a child. All these changes were being willed into existence by this young girl, who simply couldn't grow up quickly enough.

Going to the senior school was billed as a huge event for us. We were *really* going to be grown up this time, and we would meet lots of new teachers, learn new subjects and meet new friends. Sadly, my reputation, such as it was, preceded me and life picked up where it had left off when I went back to school again after the long summer holiday.

Miss Brown was my first teacher in the senior school. She was a very small woman who wore flat lace-up shoes and sported intensely sculpted calf muscles beneath her beige, Crimplene suits. She wore small, gold-framed glasses and her bosom was so large she appeared to need to lean back to stop herself from toppling forwards. She would usually arrive late into the classroom for registration and always smelled of coffee and cigarettes. Her temper was as short as her stature. She had a loud booming voice that seemed to emanate from her immaculate lace-ups and she never, ever smiled—at least, not at me. It didn't take me long to realise that she disliked me intensely, but by now my defensive armour was beginning to develop very effectively and convincing myself that I didn't care whether she liked me or not was very easy. The feeling was, therefore, mutual.

The old character trait of wanting to please my teachers was always part of my psyche but, as I started to grow up, I was increasingly telling myself that it wasn't important to me—which was just as well. I'm not sure I ever truly managed to convince myself of this, however, because on the very few occasions I did receive a compliment, my heart missed a beat and I would feel a rush of warmth graduating up from my toes and right through my body. The little girl inside me would burst with pride and I would feel the urge to break into a huge grin. But when this emotional surge reached my brain I would tell myself it was a fabrication and give an ungrateful and ungracious comment in reply. At the time, I had no idea that this formed the beginnings of a well-honed defence mechanism. I just gave myself, wholeheartedly to the contrary emotional outburst and watched as people were turned away by my ingratitude. Guilt and shame had won the day, once again.

The school I attended prided itself on giving girls a good, all-round education and set high standards in academic rigour. Great emphasis was placed on the use of correct spoken English and we were encouraged to experiment with and expand our vocabulary at all times. And how I would have loved to be able to engage in that. I was regarded as an intelligent girl with an awkward manner who *chose* not to engage in anything that required reading or hard work of any kind.

Time and again I was told I was being lazy—and so I believed it. Yes, obviously, I was lazy. I didn't know how to express myself coherently and would often find words popping up out of any sensible sequence. Sometimes it was as if I was beginning in the middle of a sentence and my mouth couldn't keep up with my brain. I would mispronounce words, omit others and get completely tongue-tied if I was under any stress at all. These attempts to sound intelligent were usually met with one of five common responses—withering, impatient, confused, annoyed or downright disinterested—regardless of whether it was my teachers, my parents or my peers I was trying to communicate with.

When I was a younger child I was very talkative and, because of my capacity to see the bigger picture, had no problem in effectively evaluating situations and working out what decision or action needed to be taken. Sadly, most of my little friends did not see their own worlds in the same way that I did and so I was simply deemed bossy and a know-all. As a result, I didn't have many—if any—close, or special, friends. As I grew older this trait became more and more pronounced and, melded together with the defensive emotional surges, proved a cocktail that shaped me into the kind of person that most people, in their right minds, would avoid. I was, in effect, friendless.

Although self-sabotage was not a concept I would ever have understood at the time, I became adept at it. In my efforts to say something, anything, that would sound coherent, I fulfilled my need to salve my tumultuous emotional surges by swearing. Although most of the swearing I used was not crude, it was vulgar and profane—and very unattractive coming from the mouth of an intelligent young girl, albeit with attitude. And now I was able to add another characteristic to the list of unpleasant elements I was developing—namely, self-pity—and oh, how that kicked in.

. . .

I was nearly thirteen before I learned the facts of life. That's positively geriatric by today's standards but I made up for it, regarding the practical application of these facts, by losing my virginity at the age of fourteen.

As I had no close friends within my own peer group, I had taken to making friends with girls from other classes and there was one in particular who was in the year below me, and who lived quite close by. Let's call her Mary.

Mary was naturally beautiful. She had fabulous, long blond hair and blue eyes the size of saucers. She had a naturally sunny disposition and, although precocious, was very popular. She had an infectiously attractive personality and came from a very wealthy family which meant that she wanted for no material possessions. I latched on to Mary and, for some reason, she seemed happy for me to do so. Perhaps she was flattered that someone in the year above her at school sought her company. Perhaps she felt sorry for me and wanted to help me—which would dovetail very nicely with my own burgeoning self-pity—or perhaps she was just a generous person who was happy to spend her time with an odd-ball.

Mary looked considerably older than her thirteen years and was the kind of girl who turned heads wherever she went. I loved being part of her world but carried a seething resentment that none of this attention was directed at me. As many young teenagers do, we used to gather together in the park or we would go into town to our favourite shops and coffee bars. Sometimes we would go to Mary's house and try out new makeup, nail varnish or hairstyles. My parents were not wealthy and, whereas Mary was already receiving a very generous monthly allowance from her parents, I was still receiving a very small amount of pocket money each week. Mary would buy a new outfit every Saturday and I would turn up in my regular kit, much of which had been handed down from my sisters. I would go to her house and— as we were almost the same size—try on all her new clothes, borrowing as many as I could without my mum becoming suspicious.

One particular Saturday afternoon, I turned up at the usual time and the door was opened by a *very* excited Mary. Her face was flushed and she was jumping up and down on the spot, clapping her hands together with glee. She put her index finger up to her lips and beckoned me in. Giggling, we ran upstairs to her bedroom, Mary whispering conspiratorially in my ear.

'I saw him, this morning … coming out of the driveway in his car … and he blew me a kiss!' she exploded as she leaned her back against the closed door, clasping her hands together across her modestly curved chest and gazing up to the ceiling. This could only have meant one thing. Mary had been walking past a certain house on every occasion she could and finally *he* had responded. Although her behaviour was no different to any other young girl whose sexuality was beginning to awaken, the problem in this instance was that he was a married man, some twenty years her senior. Let's call him Dave.

Mary lived in an avenue of houses that was separated in the centre by a small park. Mary's was a very splendid house at the top of the avenue and Dave's was somewhat more modest, near the bottom end, close to the main road and the bus stop where we used to catch the bus into town. Dave and his wife—let's call her Janice—had a young son and Mary had spent some time befriending him whenever he was playing in the park. She would fuss around him and try to engage in his games then, on one occasion, took him home when he had fallen and grazed his knee. Janice had been very grateful to Mary for looking after the little boy and invited her in for tea and biscuits. It was a Saturday afternoon and so, not uncoincidentally, Dave was at home.

I had watched in awe on the many occasions when Mary had sought Dave's attention by flirting with him from a distance, but the time came when the innocent game became a serious pastime. Mary had become completely besotted with him and, as I look back on these events now, his male ego had clearly been stroked by such youthful attention. To Mary, it was a hugely exciting game and she had no idea what consequences were awaiting her.

The relationship developed and assignations were arranged. I became Mary's alibi and so accompanied her on every occasion they met, which was usually in the dark, winter evenings, in his car. We would take a small battery-operated record player with us and a copy of Serge Gainsbourg's 'Je t'aime', and it was my job to sit in the back of the car and play the record while Mary and Dave went about their business in the front. I witnessed Mary losing her virginity to Dave and I heard the promises he made to her. It was a vicarious manifestation of my other world and I willed myself to be in Mary's place. In reality, Dave would occasionally speak to me when we first got into the car but his lust for Mary was such that nothing else existed for him while she was next to him in the car. He tolerated my presence because Mary said I had to be there. I longed to look like Mary. I longed to be Mary.

Despite our precociousness—or perhaps because of it—we were both innocent and naïve. Mary's father was a doctor and she had access to supplies of the contraceptive pill which she would take, sporadically, whenever she and Dave were due to meet. But apart from that, she never gave pregnancy a thought.

I felt a real turning point in Dave and Mary's relationship when Mary discovered that Janice was pregnant. Up until this time it had all felt very exciting—doing something we knew to be wrong, but telling ourselves it was harmless. The advent of this news sent Mary into an apoplectic rage I had never witnessed in her before. She became very cool towards Dave and refused to continue with their assignations until, eventually, he begged her to see him again and she agreed, but not with the regularity they had enjoyed before. Mary said she felt betrayed by him and began to tease him by playing with his affections and, once again, I witnessed this in awe. If only he would look at *me* that way. I wouldn't deny him anything because I would want him to like me and, if I'd said 'no', he might go off me. But Mary didn't seem to care. She pushed him away and he appeared to want her more. When she relented and agreed to see him again, she treated him with disdain. I had heard the expression 'dangling on a string' and here was its manifestation.

As the summer months rolled around, Janice was due to deliver her baby, just at the time Mary was going on her summer holiday with her family. She was not happy about going away but I said I would keep an eye on him. It was on the Saturday afternoon when I was walking home from town that Dave drove past me in his car. I was wearing a new, very short dress and a pair of high-heels I'd borrowed from my sister. Dave stopped the car and got out to tell me Janice had just had her baby that morning—a little girl. He also told me he and Janice had decided to call her ... Mary.

He looked at me for a moment then said, 'Wow, Jacqui! You look great. Is that a new dress you're wearing? Wow, you've got great legs!' My heart was pounding so loudly I felt sure he would be able to hear it. I had no idea what to say to him. I had no idea how to reply to this man I had desired for so long, who my best friend was in love with and who had only just noticed me.

'Tell you what ...' he said after what seemed an eternity of my standing with my mouth opening and closing but trying to look cool, 'the boy's staying with his Grandma for a few days while Janice is in hospital so why don't you pop round to my place later on tonight? We can open a bottle of wine and toast the new baby.'

Without waiting for my reply, he winked at me, got back into his car and drove off. After what seemed like another eternity, the power of physical movement returned to my legs and I continued on my way home. My excitement was so palpable I could hardly contain my actions and almost didn't make it to the bathroom in time.

Meeting up with Dave late at night was not as difficult as it may sound. For some months, Mary and I had been sneaking out at midnight to be picked up by Dave in his car, a little way from where we lived, and taken to a nightclub in the centre of town. The owner was a good friend of Dave's and turned a blind eye to the fact that we were clearly under-age. He just grinned at Dave and winked at Mary. I would smoke flamboyantly and wiggle my behind to the music, accompanied by sideways glances from women while drunken men leered at me. I was overjoyed with the attention the men paid me. I would be taken home by a succession of Dave's friends, but they weren't Dave so even though there was some drunken fumbling, they were unsuccessful in achieving anything other than a polite thank you, as I slid out of the passenger seat of their smart cars and trotted off down the lane to let myself in the back door of my home and creep upstairs to the sanctuary of my bedroom.

Now, as I prepared myself to go out, later that Saturday evening, my excitement mounted. I was going to be alone with Dave and it never entered my mind—or at least, I didn't allow it to—that what I was doing was either wrong, or a betrayal of my best friend's trust. I wanted to be with Dave and I wanted him to look at me the same way he looked at Mary. I wanted to be the sole focus of his attention. I wanted him to desire me. Nothing else in the world existed and nothing else in the world mattered. I walked up the rear lane to his house at around

11.30pm, went in through the back gate and knocked, quietly, at the back door. I was wearing my shortest skirt—after all, he *had* admired my legs—and a top I had borrowed from Mary that I knew he had admired her wearing. Was I actually there? Was this the moment? My toes tingled and I could feel the sweat in my armpits.

Dave opened the door and put his arm around my shoulder, guiding me into the house through the kitchen. He took me into a small room off the hallway that had a desk, some bookcases and a sofa. The desk light was on in the corner and the room felt like the kind of play den we used to make as children. He sat me down on the sofa and offered me a glass of wine before whispering in my ear. 'Isn't this naughty?' he said, grinning widely. 'No-one knows we're here … and no-one needs to know, eh? This is going to be our little secret, isn't it?'

My heart was pounding so hard I felt my ears may explode at any moment. There was no confusion in my mind. No other thoughts occupied that space than, 'He wants me. He wants me. Oh, my God, he wants *me*!' He ran his warm hand up my thigh and expertly began to remove my knickers. My body went into spasm and he teased me with, 'Is this your first time? Is it?' No words ensued. My look was enough as he gently stroked me and offered, 'Don't worry—I'll be very gentle. Do you trust me?' Of course I did.

It was all over very quickly. I denied to myself the fact that it had hurt. I wanted him to like me and I tried very hard to make the kind of groaning noises I knew you were supposed to make. Now, I was completely naked and Dave was stroking my immature form, telling me I had a beautiful body. I defied the sharp pain between my legs and closed my eyes, enjoying the sensory impulses as he ran his warm hands over my body. I didn't want to open my eyes. I didn't want that moment ever to end.

He had kept most of his clothes on and took little time in doing up his trousers while I fumbled around for my clothes and got dressed. He offered me another glass of wine and then, declaring it had been an eventful day and making me promise once more that it was to be our secret, he bundled me out through the kitchen, closing the door behind me and leaving me to find my way back out through the gate, into the lane and home.

Climbing the stairs to my own bedroom, I was replaying the events in my mind. I undressed, slowly, and laid down on my bed. My emotions were screaming backwards and forwards between exhilaration and revulsion for what I'd just done. I thought of Mary … and loathed myself. I thought of Dave … and nursed my soreness. What had I done? What was I feeling? What happens now?

When I woke the next morning I saw the blood stain on my knickers, but now the exhilaration was engulfed by the revulsion and self-loathing I had been fighting back the night before. The betrayal of my best friend was absolute. I couldn't tell anyone. I couldn't even talk to Dave about it. I wanted to feel the elation that Mary had felt after it had happened to her but, how could I? My degradation was complete. All I ever wanted was to be liked and now, everyone would hate me … and none more so than me.

When Mary returned from her holiday, events picked up where they had left off with Mary flirting and teasing Dave but I couldn't understand how Mary could behave like this towards the man she was supposed to be in love with.

'It makes him want me so much—he can't help himself, see?' she'd said blowing smoke and flicking her hand in the worldly-wise manner of Hollywood stars. Then, one Monday morning as I passed Mary in the school corridor, she grabbed me by the arm and dragged me into an empty classroom. The inquisition began.

Who the hell did I think I was? How could I have betrayed her trust? How did I think I could get away with it? Was this the way to treat a friend who'd taken pity on me when everyone else hated me? It was clear Dave had told her about our assignation. My mouth was dry, my throat tightened and I could say nothing to her as she let loose with her tirade of accusations. She said I had seduced

Dave, who only screwed me because he felt sorry for me and who had declared to her he felt nothing for me. My ignominy was complete. I was destroyed. Tears streamed down my face in place of the words I should have found to defend myself—but none would come.

Our friendship ended. I never saw Dave again and I only saw Mary a couple of times more because soon after that momentous day, it became too difficult for her to hide her pregnancy and she left school.

. . .

Soon after these events I began to explore my sexuality with an aggressive vigour that took even me by surprise. I had witnessed games being played out before my eyes but I would never have allowed myself to believe that I could risk playing those games for myself. My need to be liked, to be wanted, to be admired and respected was too great and I knew I had something that boys wanted … and so I would just give it to them. This was the way I would get people to like me. It would work. This was the one thing I would be successful at.

When I was a little younger, I used to hang around on the peripheries of a large group of kids who congregated around a children's play area, not far from where I lived. My parents would never have approved of my being associated with 'those people', as they put it, and so—

like so many other things I did—I kept quiet about where I was going and what I was doing.

It was one weekend some time after the incident with Mary that I ran into a couple of people from the old gang I used to tag along with. We went for a coffee and I flirted with one of the guys, who immediately became interested in me. A sense of excitement leapt through my body. I could feel his presence and was overwhelmed by a sense of power over him. I knew what I could give him … and he would like me. All I had to do was keep his interest long enough for … what? My brain was pulsing with electrical charges as I played the scenes out in my mind. He would want to hold me and he would come back for more. He would be kind to me. I was intoxicated with joy as I perched on my high coffee bar stool in my very short skirt, blowing smoke flamboyantly in his direction.

'Hey, my parents are away this weekend … fancy a party at my place?' I said, casually. I felt a heady mix of extreme terror and sublime confidence as the group started to pay more attention to me. I craved the attention but I had no idea how to handle it and so proceeded to increase the dosage of my trademark bad language. Arrangements were made and I waited with mounting excitement for the allotted hour to come around. I was naïve in the extreme but, like so many others of that age, saw myself as mature and sophisticated.

Around an hour after the time we had arranged, the first of my so-called friends turned up, followed over the next four or five hours by many, many more people I had never met before and have never seen since. I had planned to be at the centre of activities but found myself in my customary place at the peripheries. I felt betrayed by people I thought I could trust and felt my guts heave as my house was systematically trashed. I slept with the lad I had flirted with, enjoying his attention until the short-lived, fumbling event was over then watched, dumbfounded, as he strolled away without even a simple glance over his shoulder. I sat in the kitchen weeping. How could this happen to me? Why weren't people being nice to me?

When most of the undesirable guests had left, the person I had planned the party with—we'll call her Elaine—showed up in the kitchen after someone had told her I was in there, blubbing. She breezed up to me and put her arm around my shoulder, 'Hey Jacs, what's the matter? Don't worry, we'll fix everything up again. Your folks won't even know we've been here', she said, then breezed off again. They made an attempt to tidy up but the damage done to the bathroom walls—someone had used toothpaste to draw crude, sexually explicit images—was beyond repair. They put my mother's personal belongings back into her dressing table drawers and remade the bed. Food that had been taken from the kitchen larder could not be replaced but most other things in the ground floor rooms were put back—not necessarily in the right place but put somewhere, nonetheless.

The episode was never discussed with my parents. Perfectly understandably they asked me how I could have betrayed their trust and why I had let these people into their home. They reminded me, yet again, that they had never had these problems with my sisters and asked me what on earth was wrong with me.

'How could you do such a thing?' was ringing in my ears as I looked at the floor … and said nothing. My mind was playing my reasons, over and over again. 'I thought they were my friends', 'I thought they would like me', 'I didn't know they would do that', 'I couldn't stop them', 'They wouldn't listen to me', and the ever-tiresome, 'It's not my fault'. But not a single syllable passed my lips. I knew it was futile to say anything because I had learnt from a very early age that whatever it was I thinking, or saying, or doing … was the wrong thing. Perhaps what I *should* have said was, 'I'm sorry' … but I just couldn't.

I didn't see Elaine again for some time, but I had continued to go back to the coffee bar and enjoyed the attention of older men trying to pick me up. Occasionally I would go with them and give them what they wanted, although I would hardly know what I was doing. It would be a lie to say I was enjoying myself. I knew what I was doing was wrong, but I wanted to believe that these men liked me. At the tender age of fourteen, it was cool to be able to show boys my own age that I'd *done it* already.

. . .

Running alongside this period of rampant hormones, the awakening of my sexuality and the apparent desire to do anything I could to make people like me … was my school life. I was now well established in the senior school where my reputation for being lazy and feckless was blossoming apace and where I was experiencing dubious relationships with most of my teachers, as well as my classmates. All the old tricks of avoidance were still practiced, but now I had a new one—I kept losing my exercise books. Amid the customary comments of, 'We never had these problems with your sisters', or 'I wonder what your sister [who was by now a school Prefect] would have to say about this, Jacqui?' I just kept plodding along in my own little world.

I detested maths because I had no idea what my teachers were talking about and although I was truly fascinated by physics and chemistry, I'm afraid I was the one at the back turning the gas taps on and ducking the pieces of chalk that were flying in my direction from the well-aimed throw of my exasperated teachers. I loved learning about history but found it almost impossible to remember any list of dates. English was a complete turn-off. I could never get the hang of grammar and, of course, reading a book was an impossible task for me at that time. It took me so long to read a paragraph that by the time I got to the end of it, I couldn't remember what it was about. I had read my first Enid Blyton book—which I adored—when I was around 12 and moved on to the CS Lewis Narnia books when I was 13 or 14. When I had finished reading 'The Lion, The Witch and The Wardrobe' my heart swelled with pride because this was the first proper book I had ever read. I recall reading the last page and closing the book, then sitting for some time, just staring at the back cover thinking, 'I've actually read the whole book!'

But the books we had to read in our English lessons didn't fall into this category and, by now, the sense of feeling defeated before I even began was highly developed … and so I didn't even try. I would keep my head down and busk my way through the lessons, knowing just enough to get me through and avoid drawing attention to myself because, although I did crave attention, this wasn't the kind I was looking for. By this time, I had moved well beyond the envy stage and smoothly into loathing those around me who did well and gained consistently high marks in their exams. I didn't even bother looking at the results sheet when it went up on the notice board because I knew where my name would be; at the bottom. My self-pity coloured everything I did and every relationship I had.

Being a naturally physically active person, I played on many of the school's sports teams and so enjoyed a reasonable relationship with the games teacher—until I stopped turning up for practice sessions. I wasn't an exceptional player at any sport, but I made a useful contribution and it was the only time in the school week when I came alive. I enjoyed my French lessons and found the language very lyrical, which I think went some way to helping me understand it. I also enjoyed geography—especially when we had projects that included drawing—but I gave it up as an exam option because I didn't want to go on field trips.

My favourite subject was … biology. I would take great care in drawing the diagrams of the plant or human anatomy we were studying and because a great deal could be learnt from the diagrams only, I usually managed to get through with some reasonable marks. It was easy to visualise what I was drawing and relate it to real life, and so I could understand the information. But my relative success in this subject had the same effect as my doing well, all those years ago, with my reading test for Miss Laws.

'If you can get good marks for your biology, why are all your other marks so low, Jacqui?' This was a perfectly reasonable question to ask of me … but I had no idea what the answer was.

My parents loved me, this I knew, but I was a constant trial to them. Whatever I did, it wasn't appropriate. Whatever I said, it wasn't right. Whatever I wanted to wear, it wasn't acceptable. Whoever I brought home as a friend, wasn't the right kind of person. So I went into silent/invisible mode. If they couldn't see or hear me … they wouldn't notice me and I wouldn't be reprimanded. I wouldn't have to hear, 'You should know better, Jacqui' from my mother, or 'No daughter of mine would say/do something like that' from my dad. I remained steadfastly and stubbornly silent and was constantly told I was lazy and would have to 'pull your socks up if you want to make something of yourself'.

But there was the rub! I believed I was lazy because I was told I was but, actually, the problem was that I just didn't *understand*. Surely, then, this must mean that I'm stupid? My dad set me English essays to write for him but I had no idea where to start … so I didn't. I became invisible and eventually, he gave up. My school report cards had stopped saying I was intelligent. They just told my parents that I *should* or *could* do better.

'If Jacqui put in the effort she could get good marks'. 'It's unlikely Jacqui will pass this subject if she doesn't work harder', was the well-worn mantra.

. . .

Throughout all this time my ballet had been my constant companion, but even this area was suffering from my lack of self-belief. I had passed all my early childhood exams with flying colours but now I was getting to the more intensive stage and my self-pity was taking hold, I didn't believe I could get anywhere here, either. After receiving the latest, customary comments from school, my mum had taken a deep sigh and said, 'Well, your brains must be in your feet ... because they certainly aren't in your head!'

I recall sitting at the kitchen table one evening and telling my sister that I was thinking of giving it up, only to be taken aback by her response. 'What else can you do, Jacqui? You'll have to keep going with it!' So I did.

I decided I would become a ballet teacher. That way, my parents and teachers might get off my back. I was pretty sure my dancing ability would be acceptable and all I had to do was scrape through enough subjects to get through the academic requirements. Then I could go to college! *Bingo!*

My parents, by this stage, were relieved that I'd found something I appeared motivated to do and supported my application to go to the Royal Academy of Dance to do their teaching course. I went to London for an audition, which I passed very comfortably; and an interview, which was diabolical. My brain was working so fast, my speech couldn't keep up and so, characteristically, I started my answers in mid-sentence. Realising what I'd done, I attempted to go back to the beginning, then rushed forward to a conclusion. Instinctively, I could *feel* my answers but every question I was asked elicited increasingly garbled responses from me. When I was asked a closed question that simply required a yes or no answer, I gave the wrong one. Breathless and frustrated but desperately wanting to make a good impression, I asked if I could start again. The panel was none too impressed with my efforts but could see I was on the verge of tears so they let me calm down and catch my breath, then allowed me a second attempt at answering their last question.

It was several months before I learnt that I'd been successful and when the news did come through, it had an immediately beneficial effect. My parents breathed a huge sigh of relief and school took the pressure off— I'd managed to scrape a pass in my exams the previous year—so I was no longer a burden to anyone, but myself.

It had been an immense surprise to everyone, including me, when my exam results had come through but my mum had sighed and given me the customary response, 'Yes, Jacqui. I knew you could do it if you just put your mind to it'.

I had never shared that confidence but shared the sigh of relief. It was a foregone conclusion that if I managed to pass the exams, I would stay on at school because the prospect of my leaving school and getting a job in a shop, or some such, was unacceptable to my parents. And anyway, in their eyes I had proven that I was capable of passing my exams and so their philosophy was to keep it up.

During this last year before leaving home, I had also found myself a steady boyfriend, Neil. He was a good person and I remain very fond of his memory. He was gentle, kind, considerate and very generous. Much too nice to be spending time with someone like me … but, for some reason, he wanted me to be his girlfriend and I loved him very much. He made me feel safe and his family was equally warm and welcoming so I spent a great deal of time with them. His parents accepted me for who I was because they could see their son was in love with me.

I was happy in my relationship with Neil but craved, more and more, the attention of others, eventually going out with one of his friends—let's call him Graham—

behind his back. I was completely besotted with Graham, who found it very amusing that I wanted to go with him. Once again I knew what I was doing was wrong, but I also knew that if I ended my relationship with Neil I would be ending my relationship with Graham, so I continued in my duplicitous behaviour.

At the end of the summer term, just before I was due to go to college, and Neil to university, we all went to a party. We had all been drinking and my usual extrovert behaviour of flirting, pouting and provocative gestures, was displaying itself on the dancefloor. Neil would never get up on the dancefloor and so I danced with anyone who wanted to dance with me, which included Graham and many other lads from our group.

Later in the evening, I could see that Graham and another friend were deep in conversation, both looking at me. Graham was laughing while his friend was scowling but, enjoying the attention, I continued dancing and making sure I was close enough to the edge of the dancefloor for them to see me clearly. I was wearing a very short, white mini-skirt and long, thigh-length wet-look boots. It had become customary for Graham to take me home in his car and this night was no different and, as my parents were away, he came in for our customary liaison. After around an hour he left and I went upstairs to my room, then I noticed the lad Graham had been talking to—we'll call him John—walking up the path to my front door.

I was puzzled to see John but went downstairs and invited him in. We went into the living room and sat down on the sofa then he came very close to me and put his arm around my shoulder. His pupils were dilated and his breath stank of stale smoke and beer. The pressure from his arm told me his attention was neither benign nor loving. Graham had clearly told John about us because he said, 'If he can do it to you, so can I.' There was vehemence in his voice as he pressed himself against me. I told him I didn't want this and asked him to stop, but didn't struggle or fight him off because I didn't want him to reject me. I needed respect from him as much as I needed it from everyone else but the lesson I could have learnt all those years ago in Mrs Taylor's class, once again eluded me. I should have pushed him away, but I couldn't. I should have stopped him, but I didn't.

He pulled me onto the floor. Our clothing remained in place and, pulling the gusset to one side, he didn't even remove my knickers. When it was over he got up, zipped up his jeans and left. I never saw him again. When I finally went to bed I lay awake, staring at the ceiling, fighting off the waves of revulsion and wondering if John still liked me.

It wasn't until many, many years later, when I was working with an organisation giving support to victims of domestic violence, that I realised ... I had been raped.

A New Horizon

At the end of that long summer holiday I packed up my cases and left for college. I had just turned seventeen and this was going to be a new dawn, a new *me*. I wanted to put the past behind me and become a new person altogether. I couldn't wait to get going and, apart from brief stays during holiday periods, I never lived at home again.

We loaded the car with my belongings and set off for my new life. Mum and dad decided to take the opportunity to visit friends in London so drove me to what was to be my new home, albeit temporary, in the heart of the capital city. The college didn't have any halls of residence assigned to it but had sent a list of approved accommodation, and mum had selected somewhere appropriate for me. After battling our way through the heavy London traffic to Earl's Court, we pulled up outside of the end house of a long Edwardian Terrace. This oppressive-looking edifice was six storeys high and the room I was to share with two other young women I had never met before, was on the top floor. This was a hostel for women … yes, I could see why mum had thought it *appropriate*. To begin with, the warden would not allow my father to carry my heavy case up the stairs but my mother told her she had no intention of lugging it upstairs herself and it was too heavy for me to carry. There was a short stand-off and finally the warden—I don't recall her name but she was a large, round, beady-eyed woman wearing a faded floral dress and sporting wiry grey hair, tied up on the top of her head—relented.

My belongings safely installed in my room and my parents waved goodbye to, I went out onto the streets of Earl's Court to investigate. As I walked up and down Earl's Court Road, my mood degenerated from barely-contained excitement, through guarded curiosity and muted expectation to an acute sense of being a *very* small person in a *very* large place. As I walked past the entrance to the tube station, a guy, scruffy-looking with a long trench coat and what we would now call a beanie hat on, stepped in front of me, groped at my private parts and continued on past as if nothing had happened. In abject shock, I looked around to see if anyone would come to my aid but the eyes of all those around me were steadfastly fixed elsewhere. Had anyone seen what had happened? Did anyone care? A shudder went down my body and I fought back the tears. I felt completely alone.

I started to walk again and began to tell myself, 'this is what you wanted, Jacs. You wanted to go to London. You wanted a new start. You willed this on yourself, now get on with it!'

Slowly, I made my way back to my new home, climbed the mountain of stairs to my garret, plonked myself down on my bed and waited until the girls I was sharing my room with came in from work. I had been told that one was an English girl called June and the other was an Italian called Carla. Perhaps they would be more friendly and welcoming.

Carla turned out to be a very lively young woman who appeared to be hugely excited by everything in her life. Her English was very poor but we managed to communicate and struck up a fragmented friendship that lasted until she moved out, three weeks after my arrival. It was the warden's habit to put all the newcomers in the top rooms and so it was a sign of seniority to progress to one of the downstairs rooms which were larger ... and warmer. It was a while before someone came to replace Carla, which left me sharing a room with June.

June was thirty, going on sixty! This was the 70s and Glam-Rock was now starting to hit the scene. The Beatles had been the mainstay of the Swinging 60s but June was still in love with Elvis and most of the previous decade seemed to have passed her by. She was a small woman who appeared to have the same girth measurements from her shoulders right down to her knees. She had short black hair which was cut into the same pudding-basin style she must have had as a child in the nineteen forties. She took great delight in going through my wardrobe, such as it was, and inspecting my clothes. She even asked to try on my shoes, which were several sizes too small for her. June carried the weight of the world on her shoulders and anything that could have gone wrong in her life, had. Her parents hated her, her dog had died, her so-called friends were mean to her, she'd been sacked from every job she'd ever had and she'd got pregnant and had a miscarriage when she was eighteen. She most certainly engaged in the kind of victim mentality that put my own problems into perspective.

Over the next few weeks I took to writing letters, despite my discomfort with the standard of my writing, one of which was to Neil, breaking off our relationship. I don't think he ever knew about my relationship with Graham and he certainly didn't know what John had done. We had all done some growing up during those summer months and although my relationship with Neil did continue into my first term at college, it had been waning. Graham and John had gone their separate ways at the end of that last term at school and Neil went on holiday to Germany to meet up with a pen pal.

I spent most of the long summer on my own, reflecting on my behaviour and eating chocolate biscuits. As a consequence, my weight ballooned by ten kilos.

This was hardly going to be an auspicious start to my dancing career. My self-pity was ever-present, fuelled by the acute sense of guilt and shame I carried with me everywhere, like a badge of honour. My remorse and now the newcomer, abject loneliness, completed the picture. I was a fat pudding and most of the clothes I had brought with me, and that my father had been lugging around in my case, no longer fit. When I went home for Christmas at the end of that first term, my father told me I was, 'So fat, you look repulsive', and I reached for the chocolate biscuits … again.

When I was going to my ballet classes at home, I was the most senior pupil and had progressed further through the exams than anyone else. I was regarded, therefore, as top dog. Now, when I walked into the studio for my first class at college, I was one of around twenty five other top dogs … and a fat one, at that. My automatic status as 'numero uno' was immediately challenged as all the students in the class started jockeying for position and eyeing each other up. Over those first few weeks a natural pecking order began to emerge, and I wasn't at the top, despite my best efforts to jump higher and point my dinky little toes. Sadly, I wasn't dinky anywhere else and lugging my lardinous body around from class to class and studio to studio, was proving very troublesome.

. . .

' … and it's likely that you could be in a wheelchair by the time you hit your twenties, if you continue dancing.'

Having developed some disturbing pains in my shins I had been referred to a specialist neurologist and these are the only words I can recall from my appointment with him. You can imagine the shock I felt on receiving this news. My sister had said that dancing was the only thing I could do and I wasn't about to stop now. And anyway, there was *no way* I was going back home again. I decided to ignore his weasel words. It was a question of the lesser of the evils and I chose to follow my independence. Some people suggested that it might be nervous tension causing the pains and that I needed to do some breathing exercises. Others suggested that I just needed to lose some weight. Others still, thought I was making it up and only sitting out of classes because I couldn't be bothered to dance.

In the end, my innate instinct for self-survival kicked in and I decided to get back on my feet and work through it. When the pain got too bad, I just sat out for a while until it abated, then got up again. Some years later, I discovered that the condition is commonly known as 'Shin Splints'.

It's where the muscle sheath is not flexible enough to accommodate the exercising muscle and so periodically restricts the blood supply to the muscle itself, and to the top of the feet. So, it turned out that none of my advisers had been correct and relying on my own instinct had stood me in good stead.

I lumbered through my first year at college, mostly in a daze, wondering what on earth I was doing there but still grateful for not being where I was previously, both psychologically and geographically. I made many acquaintances but never really formed any bonds that could be described as lasting friendships. I still didn't know *how* to make and keep friends because I was so completely self-absorbed I had no room in my head for anyone else's problems. I hadn't been told I was a good dancer since I left my old ballet school at home and so I felt a strange perverse comfort in believing I wasn't. I had well and truly become a *victim* and I was convinced that no-one else in the world could understand what I was going through. No-one's problems could possibly be greater than mine—except, perhaps, June's—and no-one else could experience the depth of my pain, emotional or physical.

The physical aspects of the teacher training course were arduous, indeed, but because I had to sit out for so much of the actual dance classes, I wasn't losing any weight. Although some teachers made passing remarks about my size and my dad's comments had been very hurtful, no-one was able to put more pressure on me than myself with regard to my weight. I hated looking at my lumpy form in the studio mirrors and felt trapped in a dumpy, useless body. My appalling diet didn't help much here either. I knew that I should eat vegetables and couldn't afford to buy meat so I would go to the supermarket and buy a bag of Brussels sprouts, then go home and cook them in butter on the one hot plate that worked in our little apology for a kitchen, situated on the floor below my room. I would have a glass of milk with it and maybe a hunk of cheese then I'd finish off with a pack of chocolate biscuits. Culinary heaven.

As I had hoped, the academic aspects of my course, at least in the first year, were virtually non-existent. What we did have to prepare, however, was our own file notes of all the exercises through the whole of the Academy's children's grades, with teaching comments against each exercise; and we would be examined on this at the end of the year. This didn't pose any problems for me because I had a good understanding of the requirements of each exercise and the kind of problems you would need to look out for as a teacher. I understood the developmental process from one grade to another and so I undertook the task with some pleasure. I used a colour-coding system and, although handwritten, took great care in presenting the notes neatly and uniformly. It was at this point that I realised how important presentation is to me. As I worked on it, I was fastidious in my accuracy and uniformity, feeling a warmth growing through my spine and across the back of my shoulders as I did so. I was immensely proud of the final product and would spend a great deal of time simply admiring my work because, not least of all, I had achieved something—albeit quasi-academic. It was pleasing to the eye. It was balanced with plenty of white space around the text. The content was cogent and accurate. It was a work of art.

At the end of my first year, I picked up the brown envelope from the Principal's office. I knew it had my results in it but I didn't want to open it in case it held bad news and I wasn't sure if I would be able to handle it. I read it through twice, to make sure I hadn't made a mistake, then a sense of pure elation and relief washed over me as I learnt I had passed all my exams. Perversely, my performance exams bore my worst marks but I wasn't too troubled by this because I knew it was due to the problems with my legs. All in all, I was mightily relieved to have made it to the end and been accepted for my second year.

. . .

During this first year I had given little thought to boyfriends and, other than one or two passing acquaintances after I formally ended my relationship with Neil, had not followed anything through. I had not been sexually active since I left home the previous September. Then, just before my first year finals, I arranged to go up to the North of England to visit my sister, Heather, and her husband. I travelled up on the train with a friend of theirs called Pete, who was also going up from London to visit them. I had met him once before in our kitchen at home when Heather had been home from college with some friends, but had little recollection of the encounter … other than that he was very tall.

Pete was, indeed, very tall and willowy. He was a truly gentle giant and I fell in love with him almost immediately. He was kind, he was intelligent and he was a gifted musician. He'd had no formal training in music but he was the kind of person who could pick up any musical instrument and get a half-decent tune out of it in just a few minutes.

We had a splendid weekend in each other's company and continued to meet up after we got back to London. I had been very unhappy where I was living and, as we had been getting on very well, and had clearly become an item, we moved into a place together during that summer. He was five years my senior and I was completely in awe of him. I was besotted—the more so because he seemed to be devoted to me. I loved being loved and I blossomed as a result.

I had no intention of going home for the summer when my first year at college ended so I had to get a job in order to pay the rent. I had no idea what I could do but trotted along to an employment agency in the Kings Road to sign up. They sent me to a research centre attached to Brompton Hospital, on the Brompton Road in South Kensington because, apparently, they needed an Admin Assistant for their African Respiratory Diseases research section. I duly reported for duty one bright, sunny Monday morning, having no idea of what awaited me. I was shown to a musty room on the second floor where I was met with a pile of papers standing on the floor in the corner of the room that reached almost as high as me.

'File those in those cabinets over there, and make sure they're in the file in chronological order', a middle-aged woman, holding a pen in each hand and with glasses perched on the end of her nose barked at me, flicking her head from one side of her stumpy neck to the other, before turning on her heels and shooting out the door. 'Good morning. How are you? Pleased to meet you' I said to the back of the closed door before turning again to take in the scene.

It was a small, square room with one window along the wall, opposite the door. The window blind was closed, but there was a small tear at one side that let a shaft of bright sunlight pierce its way into the room and in which I could see a cloud of tiny dust particles. The room was completely silent, except for a faint rumble coming from the traffic some distance away, across the hospital grounds. It was the kind of silence that created pressure on your ear drums and made any sounds seem muffled. There was a smell of dry paper in the air and I could feel the dust being sucked up into my nostrils.

The 'those' she had flicked her head towards was an unruly pile of hundreds of flimsy, carbon copies of letters that had been sent to various medical research clinics in Kenya and Tanzania. Along the opposite wall, I discovered a row of around eight, four-drawer filing cabinets, each with a place name and alphabetical listing on the front. A slightly lop-sided wooden table filled the centre of the room and one, old canvas-seated chair was neatly tucked underneath it. Welcome to hell, I thought to myself, as I put down my handbag, took off my coat and hung it on the back of the door.

You need the money, Jacs, so just get on with it, I thought to myself as I buried my forehead into the cloth of my coat, my hands still reaching up and holding its collar on either side of the door peg. Don't cry ... just *do it!* I turned and took two short paces to face the pile of papers and reaching up, took the first one off the top. I looked at the name, which was unrecognisable as any I had come across before, then looked at the heading which gave the location of the clinic … again, unrecognisable. On investigating the filing cabinets I realised that there was only about half-a-dozen clinics, so I decided to go through the main pile and start by putting each sheet into its relevant clinic pile because it would be easy to go through each one and visually recognise the name of the clinic, without having to actually read the name. This seemed like an excellent idea at first, but it took me most of the morning to move very little of the main pile and I was left with about six new piles spread across the table … and nothing filed. It also occurred to me that doing it this way meant I was moving every piece of paper at least twice, thus doubling the effort. In addition, because I now had piles of paper all over the table I couldn't use it to rest the files on as I was putting the sheets into them.

By this time, I needed a break so I wandered along the corridor and found the Ladies' toilets then went next door into a small kitchen. I filled the kettle and flicked the switch to turn it on then took a clean mug down from the shelf. I was just reaching for the box of tea bags when I found myself face to face with old two-pens again who, this time, barked, 'That's Margaret's and you're not in the tea club!' at me. So, under her hawk-like scrutiny, I put the mug back onto the shelf, switched the kettle off again and went back to my little bunker. I was determined not to be defeated by such a simple task as filing but felt completely daunted by the mountain of paper facing me as I walked back into the room. My heart was screaming, 'Run, Jacs, run!' but my head was saying, 'Sit yourself down and work this out'.

I decided to stop putting the papers into clinic piles and just made a start on the actual filing but, for each piece of paper I picked up, I had to do my usual trick of singing my way through the complete alphabet before I could locate where the starting letter came. Although I didn't need to do it out loud these days, I still had to sing the alphabet in my head to the refrain I had used to learn it all those years ago in Miss Marks' class, in order to remember it at all. This then had to be repeated for the next letter, then the next one, and so on. As most names seemed to start with *Z*'s, *W*'s or *Y*'s, this was taking some time. Each time I worked out the starting letter I had to locate the relevant starting point amongst the filed documents in the cabinet by keeping my hand in the right place. Otherwise, by the time I'd worked out the sequence for the second and third letters, I'd have forgotten where the first one came and would have to start again. It was a painful, laborious process and by lunchtime, when old two-pens came back to check on me, I had filed a grand total of six letters, had papers strewn all over the table and the pile in the corner had only reduced by about the depth of my head. Not a good result for a morning's work. I smiled at the nameless harridan, picked up my bag and coat and escaped into the sunshine to find some lunch.

As I walked back into the building, bracing myself for Round Two, a younger woman passed me on the stairs and asked if I was the new temp. I confirmed that I was and she asked me if I could do some typing for her. I told her I'd never done any typing before but she said she was desperate, they were only very short letters and she was sure I'd be OK. Well, who was I to argue and … if it got me out of the bunker-from-hell? She said she'd square it with 'Mrs Prendergast'— who I assumed was old two-pens— and asked me to come with her into a spare office where she'd set me up. She gave me her beautifully handwritten drafts, showed me where the headed paper, sheets of carbon and the 'flimsies' were to be found, introduced me to a bottle of liquid paper, then left me to it.

I took a sheet of spare paper, put it in the machine and thus started my relationship with the qwerty keyboard. This was magic! This was the way I could have neat handwriting … by not writing at all. Gradually, I got the hang of where all the letters were and decided to launch myself into my task. I took a sheet of headed paper, put a sheet of carbon behind it and a flimsy behind that, levelled them all out so the edges matched then fed the bundle around the typewriter roller. I took the shortest draft letter I could find ... and started. With the aid of my liquid paper supply, the finished result wasn't too bad at all. The top copy looked reasonably presentable but I realised that in the future, with not much text, I would need to start lower down the page so that the finished product looked more balanced. Then I took the flimsy away from the back and realised that I'd put the carbon in the wrong way around, so my carbon copy was on the back of the original letter. Just at this point my erstwhile saviour walked in, saw what I'd done and burst out laughing. 'If I had a fiver for every time I've done that, girl, I'd be rich!' she just about managed, while doubled up and rocking from side to side. I was crestfallen but laughed along with her. It had taken so much effort ... why couldn't it have turned out perfect?

During the course of the afternoon my typing improved, as did my speed. I was now managing about five words per minute. Triumph! The only problem was that I was in danger of running out of liquid paper because the top copies were covered with the stuff; and the flimsies were virtually illegible because of all the double—and sometimes treble—typing I'd had to do, to get the top copies right. When she came back at the end of the afternoon, my saviour seemed to take pity on me and said, 'Well, you've got to start somewhere, girl', before adding, 'but maybe we'd better set you off on tidying out the stationery cupboard tomorrow, eh?' I realised I hadn't done a very good job and was sad that I wouldn't be able to have another go at it, but I could understand why. The problem was, I was hooked. I knew this typing lark was just the thing I needed and was already plotting a way I could get hold of a typewriter and use it instead of handwriting. I had no intention of becoming a typist and I had no motivation to learn to use all my fingers but I could already taste the freedom that typing might bring me.

The next day I was met by a Mr Morris who ran the research centre's reception area. He announced, somewhat wearily, that I would be working with him now and introduced me to the—closely guarded—stationery cupboard. I was in my element and almost intoxicated by the smell of the paper, pencils, erasers, clips, staples and all manner of goodies to be found in there. Everything was heaped together and jumbled up so I took them all out, sorted them, counted them and logged them in an inventory file then replaced them all neatly onto the shelves. Mr Morris had been bemoaning the fact that people just came in and helped themselves to whatever they wanted and didn't tell him when something had run out so I devised a very simple stock control system for him. I typed out a memo to be photocopied and circulated to all staff explaining the system then designed a large poster to go on the front of the cupboard door. It worked like a dream and Mr Morris was so impressed he gave me various other little jobs that required what I considered to be only a modicum of common sense to sort out. Rocket science, it certainly was not—but he was happy, and so was I.

When I had been there a couple of weeks, Marie, the regular receptionist went on holiday and Mr Morris asked me if I'd like to cover for her. The so-called telephone exchange was an antiquated black box with a row of switches that allowed you to speak to the incoming caller when in the down position, to an internal line when in the up position and both parties could speak to each other when the switch was in the centre position. I was pretty confident I could get the hang of this and was delighted with the offer to be elevated to a higher status— considered higher because you sometimes got to speak to the doctors who were situated in their lofty position on the fifth floor. I was given very clear instructions as to what I should and shouldn't say but, other than that, was left to use my own initiative as to how to handle the calls.

Speaking unprepared to strangers would normally have caused me great difficulty but, somehow, because what I was doing was within very clearly defined boundaries and my role was as a conduit, not a recipient or initiator, I took to it very quickly. I thoroughly enjoyed this new-found means of communication.

The head honcho amongst the doctor elite was Dr Fox and he was so taken with my efficiency and my telephone manner that he asked Mr Morris to take me on, permanently. He was very disappointed when he was told it was just my summer job and that I was training to be a ballet teacher. 'A what? A ballet teacher? What a complete waste of time!' he muttered as he crashed back out through the front door, heading for the car park. I was elated and offended all in the same moment, and the confusion between the two extremes left me momentarily speechless, but unruffled nonetheless.

When the summer months rolled to an end, the people I had been working with seemed genuinely sad to see me go. In particular, Mr Morris who, I think, had become quite fond of me. I had, indeed, learnt quite a few new tricks during that summer but I was very glad to see the back of the place and very eager to return to my own element—in the dance studio.

. . .

I started my second year at college in a very different place, mentally. My first year had been a triumph of sheer willpower over adversity, but my second year was looking altogether more positive from the outset. Having a settled relationship with Pete meant that I started to eat properly and gradually, over the summer, my weight had started to drop. Once I got back to college, the extra kilos I'd been carrying melted away, accompanied by an exponential improvement in my dancing. I was still getting pains in my legs but accepted that this was never going to change and that I'd just have to learn to live with it. Not lugging so much extra weight around the dance floor certainly helped but, short of chopping off my legs, there was nothing else I could do. I learnt to breathe through the worst effects and simply stopped moving when the pain got too bad.

My relationship with Pete was growing from strength to strength. We were blissfully happy living together in South London and became relatively domesticated in our habits. He was doing a teacher training course during my second year at college and then worked in a large inner London secondary school in Brixton during my third year. We shared a flat with three of Pete's old uni mates and so my social life removed me from the realms of my college peer group, completely.

During the summer between my second and third years, I worked in the local pub but this was a time before the cash registers did all the adding up for you. I had terrible problems totting up the amount to charge people if the round consisted of more than a couple of drinks. Most of the punters didn't seem to notice, though, and I would usually use the till that wasn't closest to me when it was a big order, so that the boss wouldn't be able to do a quick tot-up and realise I'd undercharged. In the end, I decided to leave because another guy I worked with behind the bar was sacked for financial irregularities and I was so embarrassed that it might, actually, have been me—I felt I couldn't go back.

By the time I reached my third year at college, I was in my stride. I had lost all my unsightly weight and my performance standard had improved enormously, ranking me among the best in my year. I felt a great sense of achievement, but although not particularly arduous, there was some academic work to be undertaken in this final year. The hurdle this posed required my usual tenacity to overcome. I would sit next to a girl called Jane for my History of Dance lectures and pretend to be so engrossed that I only took scant notes. In reality, the lectures *were* fascinating but I simply had no idea how to take notes and anything I did write down was unintelligible when I tried to read it back. I was somewhat troubled when it came to revising and, in the end, simply asked Jane for her notes and photocopied the lot. She had beautiful handwriting and I spent disarmingly long periods of time just looking at her handwritten text, without even reading the notes.

Halfway through my final year, we were given the first of only two essay titles, 'What is discipline and how important is it?' Panic set in! I didn't have the faintest idea how to go about writing an essay, even if I had a thought about what the content might be. I sat looking at the title for quite some time before I decided that the only way to get this done ... was to ask Pete to write it for me. He rattled it off in no time at all and I simply copied it into my own handwriting and submitted it without a flinch. Needless to say, I got amongst the top marks. The second title was 'Those who can, do; those who can't, teach; and those who can't teach, teach teachers. Discuss.' With as little clue how to write this one as the previous one, I handed it to Pete again who duly obliged and thus ended my academic experience—for good, or so I hoped.

Pete and I had picked up an old secondhand typewriter and I was enjoying practicing my newfound skill by typing out his handwritten copy of his MA thesis before passing it to a friend who then typed it out properly, in the format required for submission to the university examiners. I still had no desire to learn how to use all my fingers but I was thoroughly enjoying writing letters on the old machine and was picking up quite a reasonable pace. Liquid paper could now be bought in the form of strips that were simply typed over and so my correction process was also now speeding up. As we were coming to the end of my third year, Pete was applying for teaching posts elsewhere because we didn't want to stay in London, so I got into the habit of typing up his application forms and spent many happy hours, lining up the script into the boxes so he could post off beautifully presented documents.

I achieved a creditable pass in all my final exams and was duly awarded my teaching certificate in the summer of 1975. Pete and I had married the previous Easter and so I ended my student years as a married woman, *very* happy and wonderfully optimistic about the future. Pete had secured a teaching post in a college in Yorkshire and we bought our first little two-bedroom terrace house during the summer, ready to start the new term in the Autumn. I had contacted the local ballet schools in the area and now had one or two freelance teaching contracts, mostly working with the schools' older pupils, coaching them for their higher exams and for auditions into national schools and colleges, such as the one I had attended. I wasn't earning very much money but with Pete's salary we could pay the mortgage and what I earned would pay some of the bills. We had a phone put in and with the bits of furniture we had begged and borrowed we were able to set up a comfortable home, even if nothing matched. I was twenty and my world was wonderful.

. . .

In the middle of December in my twenty second year, I gave birth to our first child, a son. Two days before, I had been told that the baby may be very large (because the head hadn't engaged yet) and that I should put away any thoughts of giving birth until well into the New Year. Despite having Braxton Hicks contractions, described by the midwife as 'practice contractions' all through the next day, I believed what I had been told—when didn't I?—and rang my mum to let her know she didn't need to make any plans to come and visit just yet. In the evening of the following day, these practices began to feel a little too real for comfort. I didn't get much sleep that night and early the next morning we decided that Pete should take me into hospital. Our son was born just after lunchtime.

It was a very normal delivery. Uneventful, as first deliveries go and after the midwife had declared us both fit and well, and Pete had gone home to get some sleep, I found myself sitting up in bed, staring into a Perspex box with a small scrap of humanity in it. My baby had a mop of black hair and his face looked old and wise, as if he'd brought several lives-worth of knowledge and understanding with him. One tiny hand was tucked under his chin and peaking out from between the folds of a blanket which was wrapped around him like we used to wrap baby Jesus in the nativity plays at school. I stared at him for some time then blurted, 'Oh my God—he looks just like my father-in-law!'

I didn't realise I'd said it out loud but it happened just as a nurse was looking in on me. She smiled at me, benignly. 'Yes', she said, gently, 'it's amazing how old they look when they're first born, but don't worry … he'll soon develop his own little personality'. I was much relieved by her comments and thanked her as she left the room as quietly as she'd entered.

There he was … my very own baby … in a plastic container … sleeping soundly, without a care in the world. The maternal rush I had been expecting, and that everyone had told me about, was decidedly absent in those first few hours but my mothering instincts grew steadily over time. Instead, I looked at my baby with feelings of amazement—that I'd achieved it, and horror—because I didn't know what to do next. The burden of responsibility was beginning to weigh heavily on my shoulders and although I *knew* I was up to the task because we had planned the pregnancy and I was longing to be a mum, the full force of that responsibility could never have kicked in until that moment of realisation. The moment you see your baby next to you and you know that, for the first time in your life, there is something more important to you than yourself. My tiny little scrap of humanity would be totally dependent on me—and I mustn't let him down. Not now, not ever.

Most of my mothering skills came through instinct and through watching and talking to my sister and other mothers. Many of my friends would tell me about books they were reading about child development and they'd recommend them to me, but I would just ask them to tell me about it, and listened carefully. I had no motivation to buy a copy for myself because I knew in my heart I'd never get around to reading them. However, I was very keen on encouraging my son to read and introduced him to cloth books with pictures, as soon as he was sitting up and taking notice of his surroundings. As much as possible, we built up our daily routines and would always end the day with a bath and a bedtime story.

When he was a little older, we would make our weekly visits to the Post Office to pick up my child support payments and we would pick out a new book for him, then we'd take it home and settle down together with a drink and a biscuit, to read it. By the time he was eighteen months old, he had more books than I'd had in the whole of my life. I knew he couldn't actually read at that age, but I wanted him to be familiar with the nature of books—to understand that you can benefit from having books, that there's so much you can learn from them and so much pleasure to be had from them. I wanted books to be completely second nature to him and an inevitable part of his daily life. I did everything I could to encourage him but I felt a complete fraud because I just *couldn't* pick one up and read one for myself.

When my first son was just turned two, he found himself with a little baby brother. Having had one child, I thought I knew how to do this mothering thing—but my second child had clearly read a different book. They were as different as two children could possibly be, except for their love of books, stories and learning. In the very early days, as I was breast feeding my youngest, the three of us would snuggle up on the sofa together and read nursery rhymes and other stories but by this time, my eldest knew all the words—and tunes—with little or no prompting from me. As they both grew older and progressed onto proper books, Pete would usually take over the bedtime story routine, ostensibly because I was busy but I knew in my heart it was because his reading was much more fluent than mine—particularly when it came to any previously unread text, which is what most of their reading was now becoming.

As soon as they were old enough, I took the boys along to Toddlers Group and then Play Group and this is where the differences in their personalities would really show. My eldest was very cautious and would stand at the peripheries of the activity, weighing it all up, then he'd decide if he wanted to get involved or not. He was very circumspect and relied on his own judgement. My youngest, by contrast, would be right in the thick of the action, and often generated it. But he was never a trouble-maker. Rather, even from a very early age, he would be the peace-maker—encouraging his little friends not to fight and to try and see each other's point of view. My two sons always had an excellent relationship. Although there was two years between them, they played together and enjoyed each other's company. My friends would often comment on the fact that they never fought, either with each other or anyone else.

When my sons started school, my life took an unexpected and very interesting turn. Their school was very active in promoting parental involvement and so I dived headlong into it. As I walked into the school building for the first time, the smells and the sounds all seemed so familiar. But this time I wasn't a little child. I was a grown woman with my own children and I was determined not to pass on to them my innate fear and dread of the school environment. I looked around my son's first classroom and recalled my own first experience, all those years ago. His eyes, too, were agog with wonderment and he, too, chose to sit close to the door. He didn't cry when I left.

I struck up a very good relationship with the Headteacher and she was patience personified as I took up more and more of her time, each day, asking more and more questions and having lengthy discussions with her about school life, child development, current methods of teaching reading, and more. She asked me to get involved in setting up a Parent Teacher Association for the school and then invited me to join the school board of governors in the newly created role of Parent Representative. This role was, in fact, an elected role but as no-one else stood for the position I was appointed without contest. And there ... a whole new world opened up to me.

At that time, the local education authority was cutting back the school meals service and, as the school was located in an area where there were a lot of children who were eligible for free school meals—and indeed, may not have had a decent meal without it—I spearheaded a campaign to save the service. The school cook was delighted with my efforts and I started by doing a survey of all parents to find out how people felt about the service as it stood. Then we had a publicity campaign and invited parents to tasting sessions to see for themselves that school meals had moved on considerably since the days of cold cabbage and lumpy mashed potato. It was a great success and got some coverage in the local press. I spent hours preparing posters and questionnaires and took great pleasure in completing the final report. It was a job well done.

As parent governor, I was writing letters with my trusty typewriter and was getting quite a reputation for being a great motivator and for getting things done. As long as I had plenty of time to prepare and I wasn't required to read anything on the spot, I felt completely comfortable with what I was managing to achieve, although no-one was more surprised than me that I was actually doing all this.

During these five or so years, I had continued with my freelance teaching contracts but my newfound skills were making me wonder whether I could actually get a proper paid job. I had clearly discovered a flair for management and organisation and had developed an excellent track record in a very short time. I knew that my lack of academic qualifications would always let me down but felt the time was right to consider giving up my dance teaching and have a go at joining the mainstream world of work. With my customary, feisty zeal, I set about finding a job. It didn't take long.

Monkey On My Back

The phone rang. 'Hi, this is Mike. You came in for an interview yesterday and we'd like to offer you the job. Are you still interested?'

Was I ever! We had a big, excited family hug in the hallway as soon as I put the phone back on its hook. Pete and I popped a cork and celebrated with champagne that evening after the children had gone to bed.

And so it was that I found myself working as the Director of Fundraising for an organisation supporting a myriad of small charities and community groups in the local area. I bought myself a portable electric typewriter which had a newfangled, built-in correction ribbon … bliss … and thus began my new adventure in the world of work. I was working 20 hours per week which fitted in beautifully with the boys' school times. Getting a pay cheque at the end of each month was a wonderful phenomenon.

The previous incumbent in the post had not been too good at the paperwork and so my first task was to tidy up all the files. Jean, in the finance department, was thrilled with me and I became her new best friend as I systematically went through all the donor information. I created a new card index system and recorded all the donor information, cross referenced with the monthly bank statements so that Jean could track down exactly who was giving what, and when. This information was available from several different sources but it was taking her about a day a month, and much hair-pulling, tracking it all down so she could account for it accurately. Once I'd finished creating my new system it took her around fifteen minutes, on the last Friday afternoon of the month, before she went home.

I used my typewriter—and copious amounts of correction ribbon—to lay out all the information on the cards in the same format. Then I colour-coded all the different categories of information and entered the subscription renewal date at the bottom, cross referenced with diary prompts to contact the donor a month before expiry of the current arrangement. It went like clockwork and I learnt, later, that my meticulous system was still in use long after I left the organisation.

Up until this point, I hadn't realised that organising things was such a great strength of mine. I'd always been bossy and thought I knew best what needed to be done but, here I was, being paid to do just that. My ability to see the bigger picture was now a great asset and no longer a source of frustration for me. When I was planning events, I had an innate capacity to see how all actions related to each other and could anticipate the relevant impact. I could head off catastrophes before anyone even got a whiff of a problem by being constantly one step ahead of the game, and my foresight carried me through some otherwise very tricky problems. This behaviour was the most natural thing in the world to me but I learnt that others around me were in awe of my capacity to co-ordinate the minutiae while also being able to visualise the total project.

My biggest project during this time was to arrange a massive, day-long fundraising event which spread out across the whole of a university campus. This was an annual event and in my third year of running it, one hundred and twenty-five charities and groups were represented, and the event was attended by over ten thousand local residents. I was in my element, planning and directing the whole event, and I took great pride in the knowledge that on the day itself there was very little for me to do because everything ran like clockwork.

It was during my time here that I came into contact with a great many groups and organisations representing all manner of disadvantaged citizens. I began to broaden my understanding of other people's circumstances in life. It's not that I had never been aware of things like this before, but now I was coming face-to-face with it and it was a very salutary experience. I began to see my own circumstances in relation to others and what I saw was that I had had some very significant advantages, despite having believed otherwise on the many occasions when I had been unhappy. I discovered *empathy* and realised that this was a quality I could not only very easily tap into, but that I had actually used many times in my life before. The only difference was that now the empathy was being used positively, to help me understand and expand my horizons, rather than negatively, to confirm how badly done to I was feeling by believing that other people were so much better off than I was. This was a very formative period of my life and I learnt a great deal about the nature of the human condition in the face of real adversity.

But fundraising *per se*, had a limited shelf life so after my third major summer event, I felt it was time for me to move on. My next couple of jobs continued to broaden my experience of the not-for-profit sector. I was learning new management skills with each move and was gradually working my way up the ladder to a reasonably well paid job whilst developing a good reputation within the sector for being reliable and efficient.

With each new job came a higher level of responsibility and a greater reliance on both dealing with and producing written material. I knew this was an area that caused me difficulty but I also knew that, as long as I had time to absorb, plan and prepare, I could hold my own in any meeting and in most situations. My problems arose when I was unprepared for something or if I was required to read something immediately and comment on it. In these situations, my mind simply froze. Locked solid. I became adept at having left my reading glasses on my desk / in my bag / downstairs / upstairs / in the meeting room … anywhere that bought me some time. Or I'd simply say I absolutely *had* to deal with something else first and would promise to get back to them, pronto. Then I'd go and lock myself away and read through the document several times. Sometimes, I'd just ask the bearer of the document to give me the gist to save me going through it in detail and they would give me the main points, so I knew what it was I was trying to take in as I was reading it. Ironically, this masking behaviour cemented my reputation for being thorough and organised because I would never do anything on the spur of the moment.

Whilst engaged in one of these jobs I underwent what I am very comfortable to call a life-changing experience. I discovered *word processing!* Not only did this present my work neatly, always so important to me, but I could also dispense with the correction ribbons … joy! When the word processing machine was first demonstrated to me

I thought I was having all my birthdays and Christmases together. I was like a child with a new, mesmerizing, toy. Only this wasn't a toy. This was for real and would do nothing less than revolutionise my entire life … not just my working life. I spent hours and hours in front of the screen, creating text and moving blocks of it around from one place to another. Reading these blocks of text from the screen was different to reading blocks of text in a book because *I* had created it—and could correct it immediately, without laborious re-writes or messy over-typing of my errors.

My typing speeds were reasonably good by now and the notion of just *pointing* and *clicking*, *highlighting* and *dragging* gave me such pleasure I thought my heart would burst. And *spellchecking* … what can I say? This was just pure *magic*.

. . .

Once both the boys were settled in full-time school and less dependent on me to ferry them around, I decided the time had come to try and get a full-time job in a mainstream working environment. I was talking with a friend whose husband worked for the local council and she mentioned there was a job going in his department for an Admin Manager. This was just the step I had in mind so I applied, got the job and launched headlong into this new phase of my working life on my thirty second birthday.

I took the transition in my stride and soon made my mark in the department. I was a member of the senior management team and was in a position to introduce new ideas and learn a whole range of new skills, particularly in the area of large-scale budgeting and financial management. Up to this point I'd had no idea I would be able to work with figures in this kind of business environment but as long as I had my calculator and I took my time, double-checking everything, I could get by. I certainly had no problem understanding the concepts and the principles and taking every opportunity I could for someone else to actually do the number-crunching, once again, I survived.

I was a popular manager and had a reputation for motivating people and getting the best out of them. I developed an inclusive management style and believed that to get the best performance from people, you had to listen to their concerns and help them to problem-solve by encouraging them to take responsibility. This approach was quite challenging in the kind of bureaucratic, public-sector environment I found myself in, but nevertheless, I stuck to my principles and had a relatively contented and productive staff team because of it.

And because of my *can do* approach to my work, I was invited onto various council-wide working groups, looking at improving and modernizing systems. The council had recently launched a new drive towards better customer care in providing services and had appointed a specialist from London to come and develop the concept. I was identified as an ideal person to lead the process in our department and worked with Paul, the new guy, to introduce the concept within our department's staff groups. At times, it felt a little like we were trying to turn a supertanker around on the high seas but, gradually, the culture began to change and we started to see the fruits of our labours. Working so closely together, Paul and I soon became great friends.

I had been working in this role for around eighteen months when another job came up, elsewhere in the council. I considered applying for it but when I received the job details I discovered that a management qualification was needed in order to be eligible to apply so I put it to one side. But it got me thinking. I began to look at other positions advertised in the job vacancy bulletins and kept discovering the same requirement. I realised that I had hit a glass ceiling. I was ambitious and wanted to continue stretching myself and learning new skills but I had reached the highest point I could without formal qualifications.

Despite my successful involvement in my children's education, I still had a morbid dread of formal educational institutions and would never in a million years have considered that route for myself. That is, until a friend suggested I should apply to do a Masters degree in Business Administration and get the council to pay for it. I was stunned and felt a wave of nausea building up from the pit of my stomach.

'Me … go to uni? You must be joking. I can't even write a letter, never mind an essay or a thesis … and the last time I sat a proper written exam was fifteen years ago!'

She was taken aback at my outburst. 'But you know that's not true, Jacs,' she said, trying to calm me down. 'You write letters and reports all the time and writing an essay is just an extension of that … then a thesis is just an extension of that. Jacs, you can do it!' My mind went into overdrive and the nausea stopped in its tracks somewhere around my solar plexus. Could I do it? Could I? Me … the dummy who had to read everything over and over again before I could understand it? Me … the one who started speaking in the middle of a sentence and worked backwards to the beginning? Me … the one who got all the numbers back-to-front and had to keep going over them to check them? Well, why not me? I'm not going to get any further unless I've got a qualification so I may as well aim high.

I had absolutely no idea if I could do it but I just felt I had to try. The old me was saying I would fall flat on my face at the first hurdle because they would laugh when they saw my CV and the paucity of an academic track record. But the new me was saying, 'Go for it! You've got nothing to lose, except a bit of pride if they turn you down'. My heart was racing. I knew I was much happier with the new me than the old one, so I contacted the personnel department and asked them to send me an application form for training expenses. Then I got on the phone to the business school my colleague had recommended and asked them to send me a prospectus for the coming year.

I applied and, to my complete amazement, was accepted. I was told that although my lack of academic qualifications went against me, my application letter had been very convincing and my role and level of responsibility were completely in accordance with the requirements of the course. I then learnt that the council was prepared to support me by funding the course and my travelling expenses, so there were no excuses and from that moment there was no turning back. I became a part-time, mature student and could feel my wings spreading while my spirit soared.

. . .

My children were progressing very well at school and my working world was developing me more and more, as a person. Everything in my world was rosy, with one notable exception. At the very time that I was becoming ambitious and hungry for personal and professional growth, Pete was very unhappy in his work and began to talk increasingly about looking forward to not having to work any more. I felt inspired and invigorated and was reaching for all that was new. I found myself in a place, mentally, that I had never dared aspire to, let alone achieve. He, on the other hand, hated the new business environment he found himself in at the college and was very cynical about people who were wanting to succeed, progress and otherwise get on in life. He was not professionally ambitious and, although he was very supportive of his students—and was particularly successful with his mature students who were returning to learning in the same way that I was—the spark had long since gone out of his work. In short, he was counting down the days until he could take early retirement.

As a couple, we seldom argued and never had the kind of screaming fits that some other couples we knew seemed to have. I was the driving force in the relationship and, as Pete was happy to leave the decision-making to me, most daily arrangements were left to me to plan and execute. We were both completely devoted to the boys but seemed to be drifting apart from each other. We never fought but, by this time, neither did we communicate on any other level than routine domestic arrangements.

My excitement and trepidation at undertaking an MBA was palpable and Pete fully supported my desire to do it, but it seemed to become a further wedge between us. Ultimately I came to realise that we were nearing the end of our relationship.

. . .

Just prior to starting my course, that year's intake of students was invited to an evening meeting to introduce us to the business school and tell us more about the course we were about to undertake. The professor was a slightly portly man with a friendly, genial manner and was flanked by two other course tutors, some years his junior. With great gravitas, he advised us to make sure that everything else in our lives was settled and on a stable footing because the time commitment and dedication that would be needed to complete the course, whilst also holding down a full-time job—which all of us were—would be all-consuming and leave little time for anything else. He advised us not to change jobs during this period of time and to avoid undertaking other domestic trials such as moving house. He also talked about the strains that extended study can place on close personal relationships and suggested that each of us should ensure that our respective partners were aware of, and understood, the commitment we were about to make because they too would feel the inevitable effect.

We all nodded sagely and a small group of us decided to suss out the student union bar before going our separate ways. As we walked through the door I was hit with a new set of smells which were to become very familiar over the next couple of years. It was a mixture of stale chips, stale beer, stale cigarette smoke and … unwashed clothes. The unmistakable smell of … *students*. We helped ourselves to a dose of machine-dispensed, plastic-cupped, brown liquid (aka coffee) then discussed our respective working circumstances … and the prof's naff jumper!

I had no reservations. I felt ready. I would do it. It was now or never and never was untenable so it had to be now. At the tender age of thirty three, I was off to uni.

. . .

I knew I had a mountain to climb but I'd climbed them before, so this was just another one to be tackled. I bought the books from the reading list, wrote my name in the front then put them in the new bag I'd bought for my uni stuff, as distinct from the one I had for my work papers. I bought an A4 lined note pad and a new pencil case, complete with a selection of coloured highlighter pens, pencils, an eraser and a short ruler then put them neatly into the bag, alongside the books. I put the new calculator I'd bought into the front pocket, pulled the flap over and carefully fastened the clasps. I picked up the bag to check the weight then put it beside the front door so that I'd remember to pick it up and put it in the car in the morning … my very first morning as a part-time, mature student.

My first day was completely overwhelming but I stuck with it and managed to get through it without anyone asking what the hell I was doing there. I felt as if I was sticking out like a sore thumb but, in reality, I blended in very well with my peer group. There was a gang of about four or five of us that all sat together on one side of the room each week and we became great friends. This was a new phenomenon for me and I was enjoying every minute of it.

Because the theoretical basis of the course was to be underpinned by studies on our own respective work practices and environment, I felt able to contribute fully to the discussion and debate within our lectures. I was able to speak objectively in a way that was intelligent and informative and—critically—in a way that was not emotionally charged, thus avoiding my hitherto usual, trademark, outbursts. My lecturers would often tell me that my remarks were very perceptive and showed a good understanding of the issues. I loved it. I was going great guns—until I got my first essay back.

'This is an interesting, well written study covering all the relevant issues but it needs theoretical reference.'

Of course, what he meant was, 'Yes, this is very interesting but you haven't read anything, have you?' And, of course, I hadn't. I had tried—but nothing had made any sense so I'd relied on my own observation, intuition and judgement, just like I'd done all my life. But it suddenly dawned on me that this wasn't going to work ... and I'd have to *demonstrate* that I'd read the damn books if I was going to get through this. My heart sank. I felt like a big, bright balloon that had just been attacked by a malevolent pin. I couldn't understand why I *couldn't understand* what was written; but I could grasp the concepts and discuss topics at length if they were verbally explained to me.

All those old feelings of guilt and shame were knocking at the door, wearing great big grins, just waiting to be invited in ... but like hell was I going down that road again. No way! I fought back the tears, picked up my book and forced myself to read each chapter, over and over again. I looked for key words and phrases and made my own notes in the margins so that I could relate back to them and précis the context later. I got out the coloured highlighters and resorted to my usual trick of colour-coding relevant passages so that I could pick out sections to reference in my essays. This proved very useful later because all our exams were open-book and so my system of colour-coding and highlighting made it easier for me to go through my text books and create a subject referencing system, from which I could create a contents list. This meant I could find any subject I needed to refer to in my exam questions and immediately pick out the relevant passages and quotes. I was met with a few wry smiles from the exam invigilators when they saw my multi-coloured texts … but it helped me survive, so I just smiled back and got on with my writing.

The struggle to complete my work continued and I was constantly reminded of all those times I had been told I was being lazy but I knew I wasn't, and so had thought to myself it must mean I actually was *dim*. The feelings of shame and humiliation were hanging around my shoulders, waiting for me to give in and, despite my steely determination, I came close to it many times. I submitted my first round of essays and each one came back with a pass, but usually only just. And the tutors began to pay me less attention during lectures because they thought I was wasting their time, having engaged fully in class and then handed in a sub-standard piece of work. I had an eerie sense of history repeating itself …

but this time I felt I owed it to myself to get through it, to the bitter end.

Although my attendance was one hundred per cent throughout the whole course, my written work started to fall behind by the third term and I had a backlog of around four pieces of work that needed completing before the end of the academic year. Despite having nodded sagely with my colleagues about the need for stability in our lives, I had indeed changed jobs that year and my personal life was on a very rocky footing as my marriage limped to its sad but irredeemable end. I spoke to the relevant tutors and negotiated the necessary extensions then locked myself away in my room and didn't come out until I'd finished them. I passed each one but again only just.

Things couldn't have been worse as Pete and I had decided on a trial separation and he moved out to stay with a friend over the summer. I explained to the boys that I would need to do my work or I'd have to give up my course and they took it on the chin, helping by keeping the noise down and bringing me cups of tea. It was a difficult and painful time for all of us and, on more than one occasion, I did some soul-searching as to whether I was on the right path. But I knew in my gut that I was and that I just had to keep putting one foot in front of the other until we all came out the other side. I had to keep telling myself that there was light at the end of the tunnel … and that it wasn't from an on-coming train.

By the Christmas of my second year, Pete and I had been to court for a legal separation. We both put the children right at the centre of our considerations and so as marriage breakdowns go, ours was as amicable as we could have hoped. We agreed together what the legal process needed to be and pored over the legal documents together. As we didn't want to disrupt the boys' education by changing their school and I would not have been able to afford to keep the house up on my own, I moved out of the marital home. I rented a small flat not far away, so that the boys could come and stay with me at any time … which they did. It was such a difficult time for all of us, but we got through it by caring for each other, listening to each other and giving time to each other.

I found it so hard to believe that my marriage was at an end. This was so not what I had seen in my future and it rocked my confidence to the core but, somehow, when life fronts you with these things you just have to keep going and look for the positives. I knew that if I allowed myself the self-indulgence of wallowing in the negatives of the situation, my ever-lurking victim status would come rocketing to the fore and I would be doomed. I just *had* to keep going. I owed it to the boys and I owed it to myself.

The MBA was awarded on the basis of continuous coursework assessment, a set of exams at the end of each year and a final, twenty thousand word dissertation. I didn't allow myself the luxury of stopping to think about any of these stages, I just kept tackling the next project as it came along because I knew it was the only way I would be able to make it to the end. When I changed jobs in my first year, I had started to work in the field of disability and decided to use this as the topic for my dissertation but this was not an area in which any of the course tutors had any expertise, so I was allocated the head of Marketing (the subject I had chosen as my specialism) as my supervisor. I liked the professor very much and had learnt a great deal from his lectures but because of my poor written work, the feeling was not mutual. He didn't really understand how disability could be a relevant subject for a marketing dissertation, unless it was to do with aids and adaptations for the physical environment. He had little time for empathic or quasi-emotional approaches to what should be a purely academic study. But I persevered and convinced him I could do it by presenting the issues in a cogent and well-argued synopsis.

The title I had chosen was 'Marketing Disability: The Use of Negative Images of Disability to Raise Money and Public Awareness' which represented a new breed of thinking amongst the recently politicised disability movement in the UK. I used examples of marketing campaigns that had been undertaken in the 1980s for the Spastics Society (later to be renamed 'Scope') and the Multiple Sclerosis Society, to demonstrate that using negative images of the disabled condition was not only hurtful and demeaning to people who have that condition, but is also not proven to raise more money or awareness from the public. Pandering to the fear of able-bodied people by evoking a *there but for the grace of God go I* response, hoping to make them dig deeper into their pockets as a result, was not proven to work. My hypothesis was: if the marketing campaign is no better at achieving what it's supposed to achieve, and in the process upsets the people it's supposed to be supporting, it shouldn't be undertaken in this way.

Twenty-five thousand words later, the prof. wasn't entirely convinced but he said it had been well written and researched and he would recommend it to the external examiner. Thus, my dissertation scraped through. I had negotiated extra time to complete it because, by the time it was due for submission, I had changed jobs *again*. I had managed to pass my exams and completed all my course work—just—and was finally, in early 1992, conferred with my Masters Degree in Business Administration. 'MBA … I like the sound of that,' I screamed as I flung my letter up in the air and danced a jig down the corridor at work.

I had made it. *I had made it*. And I wanted everyone to know.

. . .

During the later stages of my MBA, my work colleague Paul and I had found ourselves spending more and more time in each other's company. I had found his forward-thinking approach to life, positively inspirational and he admired the way I was battling on, despite the changes of job and the failure of my marriage. We would spend hours talking to each other at work and, by now, outside of work as well. I had introduced him to the boys and we had all got on famously, and so it was no surprise to anyone when we moved from friendship into a relationship. From the start, we had just clicked and this seemed the most natural step in the world. Then, eventually, I gave up my flat and moved into his place. This was a very challenging time for each of us in our own way, but we were happy and so we made it work.

Just before I had completed my MBA, I had moved into a job in the health service. This was the period when the health service in the UK was separated into *purchasers*—the policy makers who would undertake needs assessments for the whole community and determine what services should be provided, where and by whom; and *providers*—the hospitals and doctors, etc who were given a budget (from the purchasers) to deliver the treatment and care for a designated community. My job was on the purchaser side and initially I was responsible for the development of the HIV prevention strategy across the district, before moving into a more generic planning and management role within the public health department.

I was working for a director for whom I had immense respect and who gave me the latitude I needed to develop the strategy and networks from scratch. She supported me in everything I wanted to do and believed in my ability to deliver. I could feel my professional competence growing under her mentorship and I was able to consolidate the recent learning from my course, whilst moving forward in my personal development. Intellectually, I was still being stretched at every turn but I was managing to keep pace. I had to attend many meetings and give presentations to many different audiences but I knew my subject inside-out and back-to-front, and could give confident answers to any questions that were posed. My years of teaching dance meant I had no problem with public speaking and, as long as I wasn't challenged with a rogue question, I managed to conquer my rather alarming habit of starting in the middle of sentences and working backwards to the beginning. There were a few notable occasions when I was caught out with unexpected issues but if I started to gabble, I would just stop and take a deep breath, making light of it by jokingly saying, 'Sorry … late night last night', or 'Oops, sorry … the stress is obviously getting to me'. There was never an occasion when this didn't work and usually gave others permission to tell me all about their own stress levels. Fortunately, by this time, I had managed to resist the urge to resort to emotional outbursts.

Being responsible for policy meant that I had a lot of reading to do but, given the time and the space to do it, I had now mastered the art of précising the text in such a way as I could understand, and never allowed myself to feel cornered into reading anything on-the-spot. On the few occasions when I did have to read something while being watched, I could feel the colour rising in my neck and face and my stomach would squirm with embarrassment. I could feel an inordinate weight across my back and shoulders as the writing on the page whited-out and my eyes refused to scan the text. If I was standing, my knees would begin to buckle and I would be forced to sit, then I would reach through my mind across a range of masking techniques, plucking the one that would work best in buying me some time before I had to respond. I came to think of this as the *monkey on my back* and it was a huge presence for me, but not one

I could share with another soul … not even Paul. But at least I knew I could, by and large, manage it now and I began to feel less and less threatened by it.

After I had been working on the purchaser side for a couple of years, I decided I needed to turn my hand to working on the provider side and began applying for management posts in hospitals. Having my MBA was a big boost to my prospects and jobs I might have been barred from previously were now in the running. What stood against me now, however, was the fact that I had never worked as a health professional but, undaunted, I just kept putting in my applications. It wasn't long before I had an interview … and was offered the post of Business Manager within the child and family directorate of a mental health hospital just across the northern border of the county.

We didn't want to move house because Paul was still working in the heart of Yorkshire, so I began a five-year stint of travelling a 100 mile (160km) round trip every day, but I was full of energy and was inspired to give it my best shot, so I put consideration of the additional stress the journey may cause right out of my mind. As with so many of my previous posts, this was a newly designated position and I was the first person to undertake the role so it was down to me to carve a niche for myself. Perfect!

This was the post where my management capabilities really flourished. Soon after starting the job, the management structure was reorganised and I was offered another newly created post of Divisional Manager with responsibility for the child and family outpatient mental health service and an adolescent inpatient ward. It was a tumultuous task, not least of all because the service had previously been deemed to be failing and it was my responsibility to turn things around. I tackled the project with my usual energetic and systematic approach and employed my full repertoire of masking techniques to cope with the much-despised monkey on my back. I appointed a secretary who was an absolute God-send and who was completely devoted to helping me cope with the avalanche of paper that came into my in-tray every day ... these being the days before email, of course. We worked out a system of categorising the mail and she dealt with as much as she could before referring the rest to me—and even then she'd usually write notes or references on the top which made it easier for me to decide how to deal with it all. We made a great team and I owe a great deal to her persistence and tenacity in helping me to do my job successfully.

Once again, I had presentations to give, reports to write and budgets to scrutinise but as long as I knew my subject and was well prepared, I kept the panic at bay and just got on with it. I was developing a reputation for being very forthright, particularly in meetings, and no-one would have had any doubt that I was anything other than confident, competent and on top of my brief. The dreaded monkey was still my constant companion, however, and it never occurred to me that I could have a life without it. It was so much a part of me that most of the time I simply wasn't conscious of it ... but I always knew it was there.

It took some time to achieve it but I made a great success of turning the service around and, after five years at the hospital, I left things in a great deal better shape than they were when I'd started. But I was getting very tired of all the travelling by now and decided I needed to try and find something nearer home—and preferably not in the health service.

I applied for a post with a not-for-profit organisation, back in my home town. I had known the director for some time and my relationship with him had always been very friendly but I knew he could be a difficult person and had thought long and hard about it before applying for the position. The desire to leave the health service and work closer to home won the day though, and I told myself that I usually manage to work most people out and find a way of working with them effectively, so I put my misgivings to one side. It wasn't long, however, before I realised that my decision had been against my better judgement. He was, indeed, a very difficult person to work with and our relationship began to deteriorate, slowly but inexorably.

It began with him questioning my judgement on fairly minor issues then progressed through many incidents until he was completely undermining my position. His way of working was in complete opposition to mine and I made some significant errors of judgement in handling the situation, feeling more and more discomfort in our relationship. Old feelings I hadn't experienced since my adolescence began to rear their ugly head again and left me in a very confused state ... which was, of course, exactly what he wanted. Increasingly, I was questioning my own judgement in matters that I would have normally had no problem with and, worse, the monkey on my back became heavier and heavier as I questioned who I really was.

'Am I a bad person?' 'Have I just been kidding myself all these years and I really *am* that vile person from my teens?' 'Is this where I get found out and they take my MBA away from me?' 'Am I really a fraud and everyone hates me, deep down?' His psychological bullying was becoming more and more effective until I finally realised that my position was completely untenable, and I left.

When I walked out of that office for the last time, I was so significantly traumatised that I couldn't leave the house for two weeks. I couldn't answer the phone and was fearful of speaking to anyone. Some time previously, I had bought a video tape with yoga routines and so I started to work through these for an hour or so, every day. But what was hammering at my mind most was that I knew he was popular amongst people of influence in the area. He was very plausible, which meant that people would believe *him* and not me. No-one would believe that I'd been bullied. People would think I was weak and just couldn't hack it.

Paul and I spent long hours talking about it. I played through it all, over and over again in my mind until, finally, I began to convince myself that I just had to put it behind me, pick myself up off the floor and get on with my life. I couldn't go back and change the decisions I'd made or the actions I'd taken. By this time, I wasn't even in a position to make amends. The people around me loved me and held me close, and I had to believe I'd be OK. It was an experience I wouldn't wish on my worst enemy, but I knew I was strong and this was just another of life's blips, albeit one that registered heavily on my own personal Richter Scale. I knew I would be all the stronger for the experience and gradually began to believe again that I *am* a good person and have a great deal of positive accomplishments to show for it ... including two wonderful sons, now adults in their own right.

. . .

Part of my rehabilitation involved trying to work out how I was now going to earn a living. I sat down with a blank piece of paper and wrote down a list of all the things I enjoyed doing. Then I began another list of all the things I thought I was good at, another one that included all the things other people seemed to think I was good at and a final one which included all the things I absolutely hated doing and would never do again, given half the chance. I gave each item a star rating and eliminated any that had less than three stars (out of five). I looked at the list to see what things could be grouped together and rated the groups until, eventually, I came to the conclusion that what I really wanted to do was set up my own business organising events, parties, conferences, seminars, exhibitions, weddings ... anything that cash-rich, time-poor people needed organising for them. So that's exactly what I did.

Planning the project was just what I needed to get me back on my feet. I had lots of contacts I could begin networking to pass the word around that I was at their disposal and requests soon came in. After a lot of careful financial and business planning I set up my website, planned a marketing campaign, designed my stationery, opened a business bank account, devised several office systems to keep track of money and administration. Within three months I was up and running with my first product launch.

I was very happy in this new role and vowed I'd never, ever work for anyone else again. 'At least this way, if you don't like the boss you've only got yourself to blame!' I said to my friend, who seemed to be in awe of what I'd done. 'I don't know how you do it, Jacs. You just have this amazing knack of knowing what to do, to make things happen!' It gave me great comfort to hear that vote of confidence but I still had a sense of failure lurking around in the back of my mind that was proving hard to shift. My mum always used to say to me, 'It's not what happens that counts, it's how you handle it' and I've always believed that. My mum was a tough act to follow but I tried my best and, although she was diagnosed with terminal cancer and had died as I was going through this traumatic period, I hoped that she would have been proud of how I'd handled things.

When I had been going through my divorce from Pete, I had come across the serenity prayer and it was a great inspiration to me at the time. Now, at this point in my life, I found myself turning to it again and found great strength from it.

God, grant me the serenity to accept the things I cannot change,

The courage to change the things I can and

The wisdom to know the difference.

My business grew steadily and proved to be very successful. I just handled one project at a time so that I would never become overwhelmed and this meant I could keep my hand in with other things, like little bits and pieces of management training and a few research projects with the company Paul had subsequently moved to, and was now running. The boys were settled and Paul's company was doing well. My life was back on an even keel and all was well with my world.

This is Me!

So, there I was in the middle of the bookshop, my world held in suspended animation as everyone around me busied about theirs. Could this be true? After all these years…?

Paul could see something was up but said nothing as he took the book to the checkout and paid for it along with the others. It was too much for me to take in and it took quite some time before I could say anything. It wasn't until we were in the car that I blurted, 'I think I'm … dyslexic'. Paul was negotiating the car through the Saturday afternoon traffic. He stopped at a red light, pulled on the handbrake and turned to me. 'Oh?' he asked, enquiringly. 'What makes you say that?' I told him about the book. It was as difficult for him to take in as it was for me to explain. The lights turned to green and we moved off; both of us spending the rest of the journey deep in thought.

I held the book gingerly, as if it was an unexploded bomb. I'd waited until we'd unpacked the shopping and had dinner before I'd picked it up again. Perhaps I'd misread it? Perhaps I'd misunderstood? It wouldn't be the first time I'd got the wrong end of the stick from something I was trying to read. I was now becoming concerned that I'd got it all wrong and had made a complete fool of myself, although Paul would never have seen it that way. I poured myself a glass of wine, settled myself into my favourite chair and sat looking at the cover, not daring to open it but hardly able to stop myself as my natural curiosity fought to overcome my doubts.

The next hour or so was spent in a daze as I slowly worked through the pages of the book. 'The Gift of Dyslexia by Ronald D Davis with Eldon M Braun', it proclaimed. 'Why some of the brightest people can't read and how they can learn.'[1] The book that was to prompt a whole new journey in my life. A journey that would bring me so much insight and understanding of a world of which I had always felt on the periphery.

I learnt that dyslexia is a condition, not an illness. It has characteristics, not medical symptoms. It can't be cured but it *can* be accommodated. To have got as far as I had was, indeed, to my eternal credit. I came to the conclusion that I must be a genius, not only to have survived my ignorance but to have thrived, despite it. The

---

[1] ('The Gift of Dyslexia', Ronald D Davis, Souvenir Press 1994).

book told me that dyslexia is a *gift* and, although I took some persuading, I do believe it, now.

. . .

In his book, Davis tells us that there are thirty seven characteristics that can come together in varying different degrees and patterns, which may begin to give an indication of dyslexia. Many people may recognise some of these characteristics in themselves, but where you have a critical mass coming together is where alarm bells should be ringing. When I was a child, far less was known about the condition and the two most prevalent characteristics of transposing and inverting letters in reading and writing—giving dyslexia its nickname of word-blindness—were not a great problem for me. A significant characteristic for me was, and continues to be, omitting and repeating letters and/or words. But to the untrained eye, this simply gives an indication of lack of concentration. Dyslexia is a form of disorientation and so I was being told to knuckle down and 'concentrate' on my confusion and disorientation, which rose to dizzying heights as a consequence. I understand it now but ... as a child? It's hardly surprising I ended up in tears so many times, with irate adults telling me I was being lazy.

Davis places the characteristics into seven categories covering General; Vision, Reading and Spelling; Hearing and Speech; Writing and Motor Skills; Math(s) and Time Management; Memory and Cognition; Behaviour, Health Development and Personality. That evening, I spent some time plotting my own characteristics within these categories and discovered that I display twenty nine of the thirty seven characteristics although they are more pronounced within the Memory and Cognition category and the Behaviour, Health, Development and Personality category. For example, mistakes increase dramatically with tiredness, confusion, time pressure, emotional stress or poor health and whereas it could be argued that this is a normal characteristic for anyone, it is far more acute when aligned with many of the other characteristics that come together to indicate the presence of dyslexia.

I have such difficulty putting thoughts into words that it can, and often does, cause huge frustration, which adds to my inability to express myself properly. Sometimes I speak in halting phrases. I often leave sentences incomplete—to the annoyance of all those around me. Particularly when I'm nervous or apprehensive, I mispronounce words and often transpose phrases, words or syllables when I'm speaking. All the indications are there, throughout my childhood and my adult life. I have always been acutely aware of having to concentrate very hard on speaking coherently because of my tendency to start in the middle of a sentence and work backwards to the beginning, before racing forwards to the end. When I'm emotionally stressed I find it impossible to put my thoughts—or should I say feelings—into words; rather blurting out something incomprehensible which makes it difficult for anyone to take me seriously. I *can* do it, but sometimes it takes such a supreme effort that I'd rather stay silent. My mum used to refer to my 'silent tears'. If only we'd both known why.

I can read and reread texts with little comprehension, except where I can *visualise* what is written and therefore play the *story* out to myself. As a result, text books were, and remain, anathema to me—much to the exasperation of anyone who has tried to teach me anything. It's obvious, now. Why couldn't it have been then? I found a way to accommodate my perceived incapacity to learn anything when I was doing my MBA, but I continued to believe I was stupid and lazy ... and that I didn't really deserve to be there. For the whole of the three years I was studying, I anticipated being found out at any moment and constantly expected to be thrown off the course.

I have excellent long-term memory for experiences, locations and faces. Anything that involves feelings and emotions, and the triggering of the senses as an integral part of the memory. I can't always recount a completely accurate sequence of events but I can most certainly tell you how I felt about it, or what the person was wearing, or the place where it happened. I could also tell you if there were any significant smells or sounds connected to the memory. This is because I think primarily with senses, images and feelings—not in words. I can describe how uncomfortable the chair was that I was sitting in, and the layout of the room where the incident happened. I can describe the person's face ... but I probably won't remember their name.

I have an appalling memory for sequences and facts, and information that hasn't been experienced. For example, if I'm following a recipe for the first time I have to re-read every single ingredient and every step of the instructions, over and over again. Nothing is committed to memory. Where sequence is concerned, I just don't *have* a memory! Yes, I used to dance and, yes, I had to learn sequences and, yes ... it was usually me that shot off in the wrong direction. I realise, now, that I overcame this by visualising the shapes that the sequences were making and how they all related to each other in space. I would visualise where Jane was in relation to me, and where Jane and I were in relation to Sarah; or the music might sometimes help with the visual prompts as to where I should be and what moves I should be doing. If someone was out of place or was moving out of sequence, out came my *Miss Bossy* hat—getting everyone into their correct places. I wish I'd known that this was, in fact, the only way I could remember where *I* was supposed to be.

What I realise now is that I have always thought in context. I have always been able to weigh-up or evaluate situations because I see the bigger picture. I see the connectedness of everything and so can determine the best course of action very quickly. As a child, this made me an unwelcome, bossy know-all, but as an adult I have come to recognise this as a great asset, to be used circumspectly and in consideration of others. As a child, if someone couldn't *see* what I could see, it made me tetchy and irritable, but as an adult I am learning to use this perspective wisely and in the most beneficial way. As an adult, I also have a far better grasp of the language I need to express those things that I simply *feel*, instinctively. As a child, I would be disparaging of other people's views because I could see that their thinking was short-sighted or simply wouldn't work. As an adult, I have learnt that diplomacy and tact are critically important and that biding one's time, coupled with respect for other people's opinions, leads to a more successful outcome. Sometimes, silence *is* golden.

Since discovering my dyslexia I have been able to gain a far deeper understanding both of myself and of the world around me. I am an innately empathic person but until I was mature enough to use this quality wisely, I would turn it in on itself and use it to fuel the all-pervasive self-pity I had nurtured since childhood. I could see how other people were feeling and what they were experiencing, but why didn't they understand how bad things were for me? I used to rail against the world in a haze of self-pity. I used to feel that no-one understood me—and I was correct. Now, I understand why.

Now I know that my little problem has a name, and that it's nothing to be ashamed of. I have become so much more comfortable in my own skin. I am less inclined to feel the need to defend myself. I have an *explanation,* I have no need to reach for excuses. I no longer judge myself. I back myself and I give myself space and time to read and absorb information. I make allowances for myself and have come to love reading … as long as it's not a text book!

It was also soon after I learnt about my dyslexia that I began to write. With the assistance of word processing, I had become very proficient at writing formal letters and reports, and as I described in the previous chapter, had scraped together enough know-how to write some passable essays and a twenty-five thousand word dissertation; but all this kind of writing was formulaic and systematic. It's a skill that can be learnt and reproduced as necessary. There is no heart or passion in this kind of formal, academic writing, but I was now beginning to experience a burning desire to do just that—to write with passion, from the heart; to express myself in a way that I had never allowed myself to do in the past because writing was a nightmare for me. I had always been a story teller, but most of this was inside my own head. Never uttered to another soul and certainly never committed to paper. Perhaps, now, I could begin to jot a few thoughts down? And then a few more thoughts became a story and then the story began to unfold into a novel. The sense of emotional liberation that came from this very humble beginning, is immeasurable.

. . .

So, why is dyslexia a gift? How can a condition as seemingly debilitating as this, possibly be described as a gift? Well, Davis suggests that the mental function that causes dyslexia is a 'gift in the truest sense of the word'. He believes it is a 'natural ability, a talent—something special that enhances the individual.'[2] He tells us that we are geniuses '*because* of our dyslexia, not *despite* it.'[3], and that although not every dyslexic is a genius, it's good for our self-esteem to know that our minds work in the same way as many famous people who *are* geniuses ... and happen to be dyslexic. Many successful

[2] 'The Gift of Dyslexia', Ronald D Davis, Souvenir Press 1994, p. 4.
[3] Ibid, p. 3.

entrepreneurs and business leaders are dyslexic, as well as many great historical figures. They tend to be maverick because they have to survive in a world that dyslexics don't fit into. They don't conform. Dyslexics don't learn in a linear form but we are taught that way in school because that's the way *most* people learn.

I know I am dyslexic and I believe I *am* a genius— in my own way. It's made me strong, resilient and resourceful. I am insightful, empathic, intuitive, perceptive and creative. I see life from a different perspective to most and that makes me a more rounded individual, better able to cope with what life throws at me. I have succeeded, against all the odds, but I can certainly see why it causes behavioural problems in children. I remember, as a child, feeling as if I was shouting in the wind. I was intelligent, but I simply hadn't understood information because of the way it was presented. I was charged with passion, emotion and an incredible insight, but could not express myself in a way that others understood. It's a simple step from there for a child, or indeed an adult, to vent their frustration; especially when they don't know *why* this is happening to them.

That night, as I read the book, I started to heave the monkey off my back. I was beginning to feel liberated from what was appearing to have been a lifetime in the dark. Emerging into the light for the very first time, I laid aside the shackles of my ever-present self-pity and paid homage to the feisty self-will that had got me through so many barriers and over so many hurdles. I started to breathe a new understanding, a new insight. I was about to enter a whole new world.

. . .

Davis' book goes on to explain techniques that can be adopted to overcome many of the difficulties that dyslexics encounter, but I decided not to explore these. I can appreciate this might appear to be an odd response, but I was completely satisfied with my new understanding of how my brain works and felt no need to try—at this stage in my life—to put things right. I have developed my own, highly personal, coping techniques and have no desire to risk confusing myself with new ways of doing things. *But that's just me*. I would certainly encourage others to take a different view. The important thing is to feel comfortable with what you are and who you are. What works for you, only *you* will know. Dyslexia is an intensely personalised condition and—as I have discovered—can be maddeningly inconsistent, which is another reason why it can be so difficult to identify and diagnose. I hope this book will give others the courage to explore their suspicions, and find out.

Others

Dyslexia is a highly individualised entity. As we have already discussed, Davis outlines thirty seven characteristics, but these manifest themselves differently in each person with the condition. There is no set pattern to them and the intensity of the characteristics can alter with different circumstances, for example, tiredness, stress or ill health. And dyslexia manifests itself differently according to individual personality. Where I railed against what I thought were the wrongs that were being done to me, others might have just got on with their lives.

One of the most common comments I hear when I'm discussing the subject with other people, is an amazement that it wasn't picked up during my childhood; a sense that somehow my parents should have known there was something wrong. But how could they have known, if it wasn't being picked up at school? I just don't share the view that my parents were culpable in any way. And, of course, if it runs in the family as current thinking would suggest, which of my parents might have been dyslexic and spent a whole lifetime not knowing? I can only speculate. I'll never know.

. . .

In preparing to write this book I have come across many other ordinary, intelligent people who are dyslexic and I have interviewed several people from a range of places including the UK, the US, Australia and Europe. I have promised that they will remain anonymous but asked their permission to acknowledge some of their experiences in order to compare and contrast them with my own, and with each other. Some interesting threads do occur but, essentially, my interviews have reinforced the highly personalised nature of the condition.

Every person I interviewed, regardless of when they discovered their condition, tends not to talk about it to others. This is not because they feel any sense of shame from having the condition, but because they are aware that it is widely misunderstood and they have no wish to be *judged* as having a *problem*. They know that in speaking to someone who knows little or nothing about dyslexia, an assumption will be made about their level of intelligence and, in some cases, they feel they will be viewed with pity or derision, which would be unacceptable to them.

It has been interesting to note that the younger the person was when they discovered their dyslexia, the less they appear to know about the condition. Their understanding appears to be focused around those visible characteristics they needed assistance with in their childhood, for example inverting and transposing letters, and that once mastered, the problem went away.

In one particular case, the individual learnt of his dyslexia at a very early age and was given exercises and techniques to correct his writing and reading difficulties. He had thought of it merely as a problem with certain letters which was overcome when he was a child and, as a result, he has never spoken about it to anyone … until discussing it with me. Now, in discussing the subject with him in some depth, he has come to realise that he still displays many of Davis' thirty seven characteristics and has constantly struggled as a consequence. He has always simply dismissed himself as being *lazy*. Now he's questioning that long-held assumption and is exploring further.

In another case, having previously dropped out of school, the individual undertook undergraduate study at a relatively mature age but, having already learnt of her condition in her late teens, went in confidence to the university authorities and received invaluable practical assistance in achieving her degree. Since graduating, however, knowing she would never be able to fit in to the world of work, she has engaged in a creative, individualised and highly satisfactory means of earning a living, independently. She is a classic example of a non-conforming, high achiever, so often to be found among the ranks of people with dyslexia.

It would appear that the older the person is when they discover their dyslexia, the less shame they feel about it. Once they have absorbed this new information, they are more likely to feel irritated by a sense of wasted opportunity. They are circumspect in who they talk to about it but regard the knowledge as, at last, being an explanation—as indeed was my own experience. It was a complete revelation when the discovery was made. For those who discovered after their school years, there is primarily a sense of frustration: 'If only I'd known, something could have been done about it and maybe I could have got better grades. I certainly wouldn't have had to spend so much time agonising over stuff'.

This may, indeed, be true but Davis does encourage us to think of dyslexia as a gift, and it is having these qualities that has made me the person I am, today. I struggled for some time to replace the word *despite* with *because* when explaining the notion to other people, but I am now completely comfortable with the concept.

. . .

Davis tells us that we are in good company. There are many famous, highly intelligent, highly respected high-achievers who we know are, or were in their lifetime, dyslexic. Some speak openly and freely about their condition, others acknowledge it as being information in the public domain, but do not otherwise discuss it. Either way, it sends a clarion message that people with dyslexia are not dim, not stupid, not slow. So often we will find that dyslexics are creative and independent, with unique and unconventional approaches to achieving their aims, and this could apply to the criminal fraternity as well as law abiding citizens. Our brains are wired up differently and have to work over-hard to reach the same understanding of the information presented to us—that's all.

In the world of business, probably the most famous dyslexic we know of is Richard Branson, of the Virgin empire. Then, of course, there's the late Kerry Packer who cut a swathe through the business world in Australia and abroad, in his own inimitable style. In the world of literature and entertainment we know of Hans Christian Andersen, and the highly successful and groundbreaking work of Walt Disney, whose legacy still entertains children and families today. In the world of science, we know of Albert Einstein, Thomas Edison and Alexander Graham Bell. Can we imagine a world without their respective contributions to our daily lives today? We know that Sir Winston Churchill, one of the greatest military and political minds of the 20th Century, was dyslexic. And the list of performers and entertainers, headed by the delightful Susan Hampshire and including Tom Cruise, Whoopi Goldberg, Cher, Orlando Bloom and the ever-effervescent chef Jamie Oliver, appears almost endless.

So, we *are* in good company. It was learning of this ever-increasing list of well known and highly respected people that was the last piece of information I needed to help me feel comfortable with my own discovery, and to make that transition to believing that dyslexia truly is, a gift.

Not knowing about my dyslexia caused no end of difficulty in my life. Now I know, it has given me great insight and an even greater strength to just be … ME!

Help at Hand

It would be impossible to list every resource that is available to people who believe they are dyslexic because so much would depend on where they are as they read this. A good starting point, however, is the 'Gift of Dyslexia' website, or indeed the Ronald Davis book that is referenced in earlier pages. This was where I started my journey—and what an adventure it's been. But this was only *my* journey and others may have different stories to tell.

Most education authorities will have resources for children with dyslexia and so, if it's a younger person you suspect may have the condition, a good starting point would be the child's school. Discuss your concerns with the class teacher and if you feel this is not enough, contact the local education office for more information.

There are many websites that can be reached by simply putting 'dyslexia' into internet search engines. For those who may not have access to, or be familiar with, the internet, enquiring at your local library or a good bookshop might turn up some interesting resources that will get you started.

But whichever route you choose, I wish you all the very best of luck with your own personal journey of discovery … whether you are dyslexic or not.

Lightning Source UK Ltd.
Milton Keynes UK
02 March 2010

150832UK00001B/57/P